5 Minutes to Health

**A Quick and Easy Approach to Weight Loss,
and the Prevention or Reduction
of the Debilitating Effects
of Cancer, AIDS, Heart Disease
and other Degenerative Illnesses!**

Marilyn Joyce, R.D.

5 Minutes to Health
West Los Angeles, California 90025

5 Minutes to Health is not intended as medical advice, nor does the author of this book dispense medical advice or prescribe the use of any technique as a form of treatment for medical problems without the advice of a physician, either directly or indirectly. The intent of this book is solely informational and educational. Please consult with a health professional should the need for one be indicated. In the event that you, the reader, use any of the information in this book for yourself, you are prescribing for yourself, which is your constitutional right, but the author and publisher assume no responsibility for your actions.

Cover Artwork: Douglas Yurchey
Cover Photography: Kathy Murray
Layout, Design and Illustrations: Grace Kono
Editing: Grace Kono and John Gray

Address inquiries and orders to the Publisher, **5 Minutes to Health**, at:

P.O. Box 251300
West Los Angeles, CA 90025
(310) 477-0142 or Fax (310) 477-4050

First Printing, August 1995

Printed in the United States of America
ISBN 0-9648343-1-6

Table of Contents

Acknowledgements

As probably every writer has experienced, the list of people is seemingly endless, who deserve acknowledgement for their tireless assistance and support along the path of any book's development, from the moment of an unformed idea to the actual planting of a seed, into the conceptual framework, through its expanding development, and onto the final page of the completed production.

And this is certainly true with respect to **5 Minutes to Health!** I am absolutely positive that I will miss many of my most committed supporters. However, I will pray that in their own awareness of this oversight, they will acknowledge themselves in this light, and in turn, I will experience, on some deeper level, my own acknowledgement of their contributions.

I will begin my list by thanking **Al McLean,** a deep love in my past, who unknowingly, through his own lifelong, uphill battle with a childhood tragedy, gave me the courage several years ago, to take the steps necessary to change the direction my destiny appeared to be taking. **My many other friends,** who undoubtedly know who they are, in the small city of Brantford, Ontario in Canada, will always hold a special place in my heart, for their deep insight into my need to move on to a new life, and their sincere and loving encouragement not to let anything get in the way of this change.

Of all the people who hold an important place in my life and my work, my soul sister, **Ruth Dossa,** right from Day 1, some 27 years ago, has always pushed me beyond my limits. Not necessarily with gentleness, but definitely with unconditional love! She apparently knows better than anyone what buttons to push! Her deep love for me, and total support of my ideas and projects, no matter how outlandish the rest of the world perceives them to be, has been a strong foundation from which I could be creative.

I will never forget **John and Elke Rosenberger,** who took a wayward soul (me), into their Lomita, CA home, and gave her the luxury of a comfortable, and often challenging, environment in which to experiment with her direction and purpose in life. The countless hours we spent exploring relationships, the universe, God, love, eternity and the simple but healthy attitudes towards nutrition, health, the mind and spirituality, assisted me in the realization of the need for the development of a much more simplified and basic set of guidelines for healthy living, based on what I had learned through my own journey to wellness.

And then there is **Allan Hartley,** the publisher of New Perspectives magazine, who entered into my life at the very moment when I was preparing for the ultimate writing challenge, a book written by me. His faith in my abilities resulted in my position as a featured editor with his magazine. I began writing informative articles about people I reveled in the opportunity to meet and interview. Thank you Allan, because you know the outcome of this turn of events!

I was asked to interview **Dr. O' Carl Simonton** for New Perspectives. This was a magic moment for me, as "Getting Well Again" was one of the books which had marked a shift in my own recovery from cancer. The interview was a success! After all, I asked the questions anyone who has been there, or is there, would ask.

And were it not for **Fila Barnett,** who has become a deeply connected and supportive friend since then, this interview with Dr. Simonton may never have happened. And furthermore, when the position for Director of Nutrition at the Cancer Treatment Centers of America in Brea opened up, Fila contacted me immediately. Though I was hesitant to apply for the job after my own negative experience with hospitals in the not-too-distant past, Fila persisted. She was certainly the catalyst for my next big shift!

Acknowledgements (continued)

The two people responsible for hiring me gave me something I had never had in a "regular" job. **Sandra Jackson,** the CEO at the Brea and Tulsa locations of CTCA, and **Dr. Patrick Quillin,** the Vice President of Nutrition for the company, gave their complete trust and confidence in my ability to create a program which would benefit the patients who entered the Brea facility. Their trust and reliance in me, along with my deepest commitment to the dream job of a lifetime, a job which allowed me to tap into my own background and experience, made every day an exciting challenge.

And my dear friend **Kathleen McSilvers,** who has probably brought more private business my way since we met than any other single friend, has shown me how deep unconditional love and friendship can become, despite a relatively short time frame, of perhaps 2 years, from our introduction to the present. When I, the wayward soul, had no vehicle to transport myself from the Santa Monica coast, 55 miles inland to my job in Brea, and back, on a daily basis, Kathleen handed me the keys to her car, without question or constraint, and was there for me every step of the way, until the moment I miraculously managed to acquire, with the undying persistence of the Saturn salesman, my own dream car.

And, of course, I cannot underestimate the role **my patients and clients,** both at the Brea facility, and privately, have played in the development of this book. I could not begin to count the number of times my clients and patients have asked when I would put everything I tell them into a book which they could use for easy reference when I'm not available to talk to them.

Probably one of the greatest catalysts for the development of this book was a TV show I participated in, called **Doctor to Doctor.** It was a tremendous experience, working with **Dr. Helen Pensanti,** the interviewer, and **Barbara Hoffman,** the producer. I acknowledge these two special individuals for their commitment to making a difference in the health of their fellow humans, as well as their endless, and at times, stretched patience with me, through all of the unforeseen setbacks which arose during the process of the production of this labor of love.

When it came to the cover for this book, I had a concept. Somehow I seemed unable to convey this concept to an artist. I had almost given up hope of seeing my vision become a reality, when into my life, thanks to my dear and loyal friend **Venetia Featherstone-Witty,** came **Doug Yurchey.** Though I gave him very little to work with, I almost fell over with shock when he presented to me my original concept for the cover. I had not shared this particular concept with him!

I could not complete this section without a very special thanks to **Grace Kono,** at Keystrokes in Santa Monica. Not only the fastest typist I know, but also the most inventive and thorough at her job. She took a basic manuscript and made it interesting and unique from a reader's perspective. And on top of everything, she was there for me every step of the way!

And finally, a special thanks to some very important people for their tremendous belief in me at times when even I had lost faith in the project. The brevity of description of the following individuals in no way diminishes the value or essential nature of their contribution and relationship to the final outcome of this completed work. If it were not for their unconditional love, support, strength and relentless lessons, I doubt there would have been a book entitled **5 Minutes to Health!** At least not by Marilyn Joyce.

The list includes the following: **Nancy Newman** (my deceased friend and client), **Irene Newman** (her mother and my friend), **Mary Burt,** my Mother (who I long to be friends with on mutual terms), **John Gray** (my special love and confidant), **Randall Leonard** (whose music and soul lifted me from hell!), **Terry Braverman** (who has continually sparked my growth with humor), **Nelson Jervis** (who always remembers to call at my lowest moments), **Karen Connelly** (whose door was always open at any hour of the day or night for the wandering wayward soul searching for the answers to life and God!), **Susan Chedu** (my special and very much loved stepdaughter who never forgets to call and express her love and keep the lines of communication open), **Dan McGuin** (the gatekeeper for all of my past possessions and a long term supporter of any dreams I dare to dream), **Dr. Gloria Phillips and Hope Pliskow** at California Medical Arts (who have continually believed in, and supported my work, referring many clients to me), **Zann Lascot** (whose deep conviction to my success has pushed me forward despite myself), **Jerry Rowitch** (who, due to his faith in me and belief in my potential, when I was still lost in the woods, assisted the opening of many critical doors), **Kerk Brown** (one of the few bank managers I know with heart and understanding), **Melonie Burke** (the first person to really help me get to the route of my deepest fears and move closer to the truest sense of myself I have ever realized), **Larry Eckstein,** the past Medical Director at California Medical Arts (whose friendship and confidence in my work meant more to me than I can put into words -- the break he provided for me was the start of a renewed belief in my career choice!), **Randy Ripley** (who has no mercy when he cajoles me into moving forward in my projects without excuses), **Robert Beechy** (my long time friend who saw very clearly, many years ago, what direction my life needed to take, and quietly supported me through all of the emotional turmoil I encountered on the long road to change and progress), **Martin Rutte and Tim Clauss** (who both, with love and compassion, opened my soul many years ago, to the great potential I had locked up inside of myself), **Suzanne Taylor** (whose continued love and respect for me has never depended on anything but who I really am on the deepest levels), **Patti Leviton** (a new and dear friend, who has supported my work and my soul, through the many unexpected challenges over the past year) and finally, **Kathy Murray** (the most endearing photographer I have ever worked with, who so unquestionably believed in my work, that she devoted her personal time to producing the most realistic, yet beautiful shots, of me, for my promotional packages and the cover of this book).

And to all of those I have forgotten to mention, thank you so much for everything you have contributed to the completion of **5 Minutes to Health!**

- Foreword -

Why Such a Book by Marilyn Joyce?

In 1984, I, Marilyn Joyce, had the world by the tail! Or so it seemed! On the surface, everything looked like it was working. I had my own nutrition consulting business, demanding a high fee for my services. I was living in a beautiful home which I owned, driving the car of my dreams, traveling extensively, dating a number of very successful men in the business world, and was basically writing my own ticket in every aspect of my life.

My peers, my employers, my clients and my audiences alike, had nothing but good things to say about my work and my pleasant, friendly, accommodating (people pleasing) nature! I would bend over backwards to make sure that I had covered every possible detail, and more, in the name of my work. It was not uncommon for me to work around the clock for days on end in order to meet unrealistic deadlines. My resume was full of letters from satisfied clients stating that, "Marilyn always gives at least 130% to every challenge she is faced with." But, after all, this business was my baby, and that's what one had to do to get ahead! Or so I thought!

For about two years, I rode the crest of that wave, and thought I loved every moment of it. Though I did spend a lot of time marvelling at my seemingly great success. And spent many sleepless nights wondering how I had managed to pull this off, and how long it would last before something would bring it to a crashing halt. You see, I did not really enjoy the feeling of success! I was too busy worrying about it coming to an end!

And end it did! Suddenly my world shattered around me. My business contracts, which were primarily government-based, ended overnight, with sudden cutbacks in spending in the particular arena of my focus. My car was totalled in the first major accident of my driving career. Somehow, I, and my friends, who were in my car at the time, were only slightly bruised, if at all. However that did not deter a lawsuit by one of my passengers. A nasty ending to a so-called friendship!

There's more! One of my closest friends, for reasons unknown, committed suicide a week later. Her business was at its greatest height of success at that time! And we, her closest friends, all envied her wonderful marriage to one of the most loving, demonstrative men we had ever known! Something in this picture did not fit!

What appeared to be unfolding into the relationship of my dreams, ended about the same time as the suicide occurred. One day we were speaking about marriage. The next day, without any explanation, "the love of my life", called the whole thing off!

And, of course, as a result of this whole sequence of events, I was faced with a monthly mortgage that was, now, beyond my limits. So I had to begin the process of selling my beautiful home with all of the amenities I so enjoyed. I knew it couldn't get worse than this! After all, nothing that I had worked so long and so hard for, was still available to me.

Wrong! To coin a phrase, what happened next was, literally, the straw that broke the camel's back!! An unusual looking, hard black mole appeared on my face. My vanity took me to the doctor. The shock of the diagnosis sent me spinning. Melanoma! On my face and my back! I'm sure you could have knocked me over with a feather.

However, I was assured that we got it early, and that there was probably no cause for concern. Out of hospital a week, I was rushed back into the hospital, with tremendous pain in my uterus. You can probably guess by now what the diagnosis was.

Here I was 36 years old, and given a death sentence. After all, in every hospital or nursing home I worked in, the moment a patient or resident was diagnosed with any kind of cancer, we began preparing them for "the end," in other words, DEATH! It is not uncommon to hear a doctor or a nurse state that "It's only a matter of time!" And I had bought into that belief, hook, line and sinker, so to speak. Who was I to believe that my odds were any better than anyone else's?

Was I depressed? You're darn right I was! Did I show it? Not a chance! The world was only going to see me at my best. By this point in my life, it was ingrained in me that I must never let anyone see my vulnerabilities, my weaknesses. I was known as a survivor, by most people who knew me, and as well, I was a Dietitian, who talked about health and how to achieve it. It was critical that I put up a good front, until the bitter end. If people were aware of my condition, I would lose my credibility!

Several years into my struggle with cancer, someone in a nowhere town in mid-somewhere USA, really summed up the story of my life, at least until that point in time: "Lookin' good! That's all you care about, Marilyn! Your only concern is what you and your life look like to the onlooker! Make sure you don't let anyone get too close now, just in case they get to know who you really are." So you might say that I was at an impasse in my life and with my illness.

Without going into the details of my illness, suffice it to say I went progressively down hill. At the point at which I was not given a lot of time, the realization that "Lookin' good!" was not cutting it, hit like a lightning bolt! I was not looking good! And the myriad of excuses I used to explain my tremendous weight loss and extreme fatigue, were growing old, and not very believable.

I had tried everything! Every diet and every program I could find or stumble upon. Every idea anyone suggested. Every vitamin and mineral written about in the literature, whether scientific, or popular. Every herb and every tea anyone talked about. And my personal library of books and information filled every shelf in my home and covered every available space on my floors. And let's not forget that I was a trained dietitian with a major emphasis on biochemistry. If anyone should have the answers, I should! Right?

Well, if I had remembered my biochemistry, I might have had some answers sooner. However, cancer, like all illnesses, is a teacher. And my lesson was about learning to listen. It was obvious that I did not have all of the answers. Yet, in my effort to hide my own problem, I would attempt to have a solution for everyone else's problem, and avoid dealing with my own situation. Of course, the day of reckoning always arrives! And fortunately it saved my life!

A homeshow, a Vita-Mix machine, a young man knowledgeable about things I had forgotten about, and a Bernie Siegel workshop. *Love, Enzymes and Miracles!* (My own summation of this cummulative set of events.) As I began to research and remember about enzymes in food, and the need for that food to be alive and wholesome, filled with all the nutrients necessary for the biochemical functions of my body, I saw the need for a drastic change. From foods that simply provided calories, to foods that had a lot more than calories and fat to offer.

With a lot of help from a couple of devoted and true friends, and the implementation of very basic and quick-to-prepare recipes, my health began to improve. The focus was mainly on raw foods in more bioavailable forms. A wide variety of fresh vegetables and wholegrains formed the basis of my diet, with the addition of a little fruit and a small portion of fish every day. I added green things, such as spirulina, barley grass, chlorella, various seaweeds, and an all-natural protein powder called Super-Green Pro-96, by Nature's Life.

To begin with, I had almost no energy to even eat. However, little by little, I was able to consume more, primarily in liquid forms. Using a Vita Mix-Machine, which is a high-powered blender, food processor, grinder, grater, chopper and mixer all rolled into one machine, I got all of my foods in the whole food state, but in a much more bioavailable or digestible form. Within a month, I was able to tolerate more solid foods. Just for the record, I have continued to use a Vita-Mix machine simply because of the speed with which a delicious wholesome meal can be prepared.

As well, I realized throughout my own healing process, that the most productive practices I employed, were also generally the simplest, least time-consuming practices! Whether they involved the physical, mental or spiritual aspects of getting well again, *simplicity* appeared to be the key.

Since my recovery, I have continued to incorporate the 80-20 principle, whereby my diet is predominantly free of over-processed and over-prepared foods. Once in a while, when I go out with friends, I may indulge in foods which are not as close to natural as the foods I eat at home. But "fast food" is not on my menu! And left to my own devices, I will choose a restaurant which serves a variety of healthy food choices, versus the opposite. I steer clear of the rich desserts and items prepared with heavy cream sauces.

In my work with clients and patients, it became evident to me that those who incorporated a similar pattern of simple healthy eating and lifestyle habits, began to see major improvements in their health. Getting back to basics seems to be the key to good health! The minute we move away from a simple lifestyle, we begin to complicate our lives and to create tremendous stress on our bodies, which in time, leads to a breakdown of our immune systems. And then our bodies, in turn, fall prey to an attacking illness.

So you see, this book is the result of dealing with my own illness, as well as my work with a wide variety of degenerative illnesses in my nutrition and lifestyle practice. It is at the request of my clients and patients, to put all of the basics into a form that they can refer to at any time, that this book became a reality!

It is important to state here, that when it comes to illness, there are no magic bullets. There is no one thing that will be the answer for everyone. But a simple, high quality diet and lifestyle regime will, at least, give a person a fighting chance. For a more individualized program, designed specifically for you, it is important to seek out reliable, credible professionals to work with you.

Furthermore, be assertive! Take nothing at face value. Ask questions. Become involved, and be a participant in your healing process. Choose health and wellness over illness! Choose quality over quantity. Choose natural, whole foods over processed, denatured foods. Choose simplicity over complexity. Choose to be self-reliant, taking responsibility for your own care, versus depending on your doctor or other healthcare providers to "make" you well again. Seek out the kind of support you need and use it. See your illness as your teacher, your friend, and pay attention to what it is trying to tell you.

Most importantly, think of this road that you are about to travel on, as an adventure. It is an opportunity to explore your options and to try new approaches to the way you live your life. It is your chance to take charge of your body and your life.

With love, I offer this book, to assist you in making some of the changes necessary to insure your continued health, or to overcome a life-threatening illness, should that be the journey you happen to find yourself on at this time.

I will also leave you, at this point, with two statements I have adopted into my consciousness as a result of my own journey to wellness.

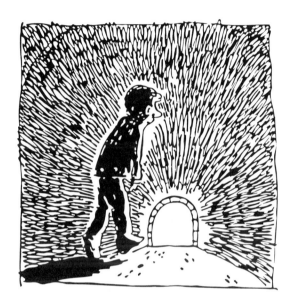

"If it doesn't flow, it doesn't go!"

And remember:

> **"It ain't over `till it's over!"**

Marilyn Joyce, R.D.
5 Minutes to Health
P.O. Box 251300
West Los Angeles
California 90025

Why a Book Called "5 Minutes to Health"?

In our modern existence we bend over backwards to create a simpler, more convenient and efficient environment, in which the flow of our lives is unencumbered by a series of monotonous tasks and activities, such as housework and cooking. We have machines for every task! Of course the thought of the upkeep, maintenance and cleaning of the equipment is enough to have us running out to the nearest fast food establishment for most of our meals!

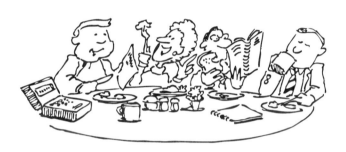

The fact is, however, with a gadget for every job, we hardly know where to start or what to use. The confusion halts us in our tracks. The fear of cleanup alone stops the equipment from making it out of the cupboard and onto the shelf. The common lament that I hear from my clients, and the population in general, is that it takes just too much time and effort to prepare healthy food. This thought alone stops the process of preparation!

As if that thought by itself was not enough of a deterrent to the implementation of healthy eating habits, the other most common reason expressed for continuing to purchase convenience foods and fast food meals, is the supposed expense of buying healthy foods, such as fresh fruits and vegetables and natural unprocessed grains and protein sources.

Working in the field of health and fitness for the past 27 years, the latter 15 years as a dietitian, primarily in private practice, and working in conjunction with a variety of health and fitness centers, as well as institutions for care of the ill or infirmed populations, it became clear to me that most people do not have a clue as to how simple it is to create health in their lives on a consistent basis. In their frustration weeding through text, after complicated text, most of which address the *why* instead of the *how-to*, they give up and return to, or continue their old, generally unhealthy nutrition and lifestyle patterns. Their excuse: *It is too complicated to figure out what to do to be healthy!*

In my work with my clients and patients, I outline the various strategies and techniques required to effectively reach and maintain health and vitality. At their request, I go into their homes and, literally, empty out their refrigerators and cupboards of all of the health-robbing processed items taking up the space required for nutritious and life-supporting foods. We then shop, and stock their kitchens with the highest quality foods and condiments available, purchased from the best sources in their area. We evaluate and simplify the amounts and types of equipment used, as well as the methods of food preparation incorporated. And finally, I provide a variety of easy, quick recipes to get started with.

Within weeks, even days, I receive calls telling me how much better, not only my patient is feeling, but also the rest of the family or household members!

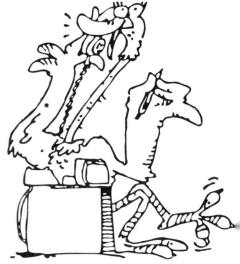

Over the years, my clients, patients and friends have asked me to put these guidelines and recipes into a form that they can refer to at any time, instead of having to call me every other day for ideas or confirmation that what they are doing is correct or appropriate. Hence, the reason for this book!

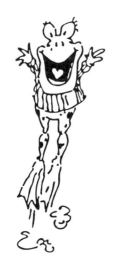

5 Minutes to Health is going to show you, the reader, that being healthy and eating nutritious foods is absolutely no more expensive, if as expensive, as eating all of those convenience foods which are so available. And which seem to be so appealing, thanks to the efforts of diligent advertising agents who have little or no knowledge of, or interest in, nutrition. But who have a tremendous vested interest in a wide profit margin! *Remember, advertisements are for profit only, not for your health!*

This book will show you how simple and quick good nutrition, leading to sound health, can be. This is a *How-To* manual! There are no tricks to being healthy. Just simple, straight forward techniques, which take little or no effort to incorporate into your life on a consistent daily basis. *The goal here is to dispell the myths that you have to be rich to be healthy, and that only those who have the luxury of time can achieve optimum health.*

With only a few minutes a day, and a well setup kitchen, with only the most necessary equipment and utensils, and the most appropriately stocked pantry and refrigerator, anyone can achieve enviable health and vitality!

Every effort has been made to put the information in this manual into a simple format, which is easy-to-follow and incorporate. Lists and charts are used whenever feasible, so that the reader may easily make copies of these to place in appropriate places for reference, such as a refrigerator or cupboard door.

As much as possible, choice -- your choice -- has been an important aspect of this book's contents. Choice of specific meals. Choice of the foods selected. Choice of the amount and types of seasonings used. Because most of us feel often that we have so little control over the various aspects of our lives, it is very important for us to have a sense of control and choice with respect to what we put into our bodies. Generally, we just need the facts, the directions, and some useful ideas, to get started on the exciting and adventurous, and sometimes challenging, journey towards optimum health. My deepest desire is that this book will entice you into joining me on this wonderful trip through life on the road to fun and adventure in the abundant world of tasty and appetizing delights!

So, are you ready to begin? Okay, let's hit the road!

The Rules for the Road

It's actually pretty simple. If you want to be healthy and alive, you have to get foods with a life of their own into your body. So the following rules for the journey towards health and a vibrant life are very logical. We will begin on a positive note, with a list of only the DO's.

1. **Select the freshest foods you can find!** As food sits for long periods of time it becomes:

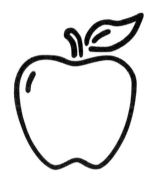

    a.   stale with poor flavor, texture and appearance,

    b.   rancid if it contains oils (grains, nuts, seeds),

    c.   depleted of nutrients which are destroyed by exposure to oxygen in the air.

2. **Focus on fresh vegetables and fruits, and raw untoasted, unroasted grains and cereals.**

3. *Look for reliable sources,* either within your area, or by mail order, for **organic produce and grains,** and use these as much as possible in your daily menus. *Seek out the local or closest farmers' market* and shop there for produce.

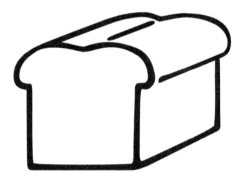

4. **Use the simplest, shortest cooking methods possible** when preparing your food in order to insure optimum retention of nutrients. In other words, steam vegetables only to the point of el dente, grill fish and chicken until just done, steam rice or grains until tender and then remove from heat immediately. Gently simmer on low heat versus rapidly boiling on a high heat.

5. Aim to eat at least 50% of your vegetables and fruits in their raw form. This preserves the vitamins, minerals and active enzymes, which may be destroyed by heat and water during the cooking process. Your body requires a full profile of all of these nutrients, which work together, when in proper balance, to create the potential for every metabolic function within the body to take place.

6. Eat the skins of your produce items (fruits and vegetables) whenever possible. Many of the essential nutrients are right under the skin.

7. Choose whole vegetables and fruits over their juices. The fiber which is discarded in the production of the juice is very high in vitamins, minerals and phytochemicals (plant chemicals), all of which are essential in the prevention of disease and illness. The juice contains only a portion of what is available in the whole food!

8. Season foods with natural condiments, such as fresh herbs, fresh garlic, onions, lemon or lime juice, peppers, organic and ethnic vinegars, vegetable flakes and powders, and spices.

9. Include a wide variety of foods in your diet. This insures a better balance of essential nutrients. What one food lacks, another contains!

10. Reduce your intake of fats, especially saturated fats. These include fats from dairy products and most animal protein sources, other than fish and seafood.

11. Use methods of cooking which do not require the addition of fats, or substitute the fats with vegetable broth, water, or fresh lemon juice.

12. Include small amounts of fats in your diet which are from plant oil sources, focusing on pure virgin olive oil, canola oil and sesame oil. Use them uncooked, in dressings, for salads and steamed vegetables.

13. Steer clear of any fats which are of a trans-fatty acid nature, or which incorporate hydrogenation in the processing. These include:

- the wide array of margarines
- salad dressings
- mayonnaise
- most commercial nut butters (eg. peanut butter)
- roasted nuts and seeds
- packaged and frozen baked goods, cookies, crackers
- snack foods and snack bars
- canned, packaged and frozen entree items
- powdered, canned, refrigerated or frozen coffee whiteners
- powdered flavored coffee mixes
- non-diary creams and dessert toppings

In other words, check the label for the words *hydrogenated,* or *partially hydrogenated,* or *palm oil,* or *coconut oil,* or *any other oil which is listed as hydrogenated.* Leave it on the shelf or in the case. These do not spell good health!

14. Reduce or eliminate your consumption of meats, especially red meats (ie. beef, pork, lamb). These meats are high in marbled saturated fats. Apart from the health risks associated with high fat intake, as indicated throughout the research, the fat of the animal is also where the toxic byproducts of metabolism, and the hormonal injections for faster growth, are stored.

15. Choose fish or the leaner cuts of poultry, ie. the chicken or turkey breast *with the skin removed, in place of red meats.* If using ground turkey meat, select the skinless boneless breast of the turkey and ask the butcher to grind it for you.

16. Game meat provides a very lean and tasty alternative to our higher fat domestic protein sources. These include rabbit, hare, muskrat, deer, moose, caribou, bear, wild goose, grouse, pheasant, turtle, frog legs, rattlesnake and eels, just to mention a few.

17. Limit your intake of animal meats to a maximum of 3 to 5 servings per week, with the focus on the leaner varieties, especially fish. Fish is generally high in a type of oil, commonly referred to as omega-3 fish oil, which appears to be beneficial in the reduction of the incidence of heart disease and various cancers.

18. Select the plain, unflavored, nonfat and lowfat versions of dairy products, such as milk, cottage cheese, ricotta cheese, buttermilk and yogurt. Look for the lower fat varieties, now available, of firm cheeses. Or better still, *try some of the new soy cheeses in the dairy section* of the grocery store or health food store.

19. Increase your consumption of legumes as a high fiber, low fat, high calcium and iron source, of protein. Included are soybeans and soybean products, such as tempeh, tofu, miso, and soymilk. Other varieties of legumes: chickpeas (garbanzo beans), pinto beans, white and red kidney beans, Roman beans, split peas, lentils, black-eyed peas, etc.

20. Include at least 2 cups of plain, nonfat yogurt, kefir, or acidophilus milk daily for their immune-enhancing properties. Select only those brands which list the specific cultures, and list them as *Live Cultures*.

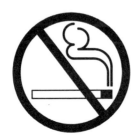

21. Reduce or eliminate the intake of potential toxins.

Tobacco has been associated with illnesses and diseases too numerous to list here.

Alcohol can lead to illnesses of the liver, kidneys, bladder and overall elimination systems of the body.

Pesticides on our fresh produce may have hazardous effects on our overall health and immune systems. It is advisable to wash all produce upon purchase, even if it is organically grown. Add 1/2 cup of white vinegar to a basin of clean purified water, and soak produce, other than berries and leafy greens, for several minutes, and then rinse thoroughly in two sinks of clear water. Let dry on towels and then refrigerate.

Additives and preservatives added to our food sources may prove over time to have deleterious effects on our immune systems and general well-being. With the increasing consumption of packaged, processed preserved foods we are also seeing a parallel in increasing numbers of allergy sufferers, and general lethargy and restlessness among our children and adolescents. Is there a connection? Why take the risk?

22. Minimize risky foods. These include:

- fatty meats
- salty foods
- sugar-laden desserts, chocolates and sweets
- pickled foods, especially those produced with white, distilled vinegar
- salt-cured meats and foods
- smoked meats, cheeses and other foods
- nitrite-cured meat products and other foods
- burned or well-done foods, including and especially those cooked on a barbecue

23. Daily intake of fluids should include at least 6 to 8, 8 ounce glasses of water. The diet in this book is high in natural fiber, which absorbs, like a sponge, many times its own weight in fluids. Without adequate fluid intake, you can become severely constipated, as well as experience flatulence (gas) and bloating.

Water is required for every major function of the body, including carrying nutrients to where they are needed, as well as carrying wastes and toxins out of the body. Water is also necessary for proper functioning of the digestive juices and the digestive tract, so it may assist in prevention of indigestion.

If you are ill, it is advisable to increase your fluid intake, to prevent dehydration which can result from diarrhea, vomiting, high fevers or hyperventilation.

24. Regular daily exercise is essential for maintenance of an efficient, fully functioning and energized body. However, *gentle exercise,* done consistently, is the key to long term benefits. This includes natural forms of exercise, such as walking, swimming, climbing stairs (versus taking the elevator or escalator), bicycling, dancing, yoga and sexual activities.

Love your body with exercise. Gentle exercise is nurturing and soulfully nourishing. Punishing forms of exercise are breaking down tissue which then has to be rebuilt! *If you are ill, you do not have the extra stores* for any additional rebuilding, over and above the extra demanded for basic maintenance!

25. Respect and Love this wonderful machine: Your Body!

Listen to it! Be alert to any signals of *dis-ease,* indicating that something is not working right in the body. These can include pain in a part or parts of the body, indigestion, heartburn, constipation, diarrhea, flatulence, vomiting, fatigue, anxiety, irregular hair or nail growth, excessive fluid retention, or bloating, just to mention a few.

So to sum up what you have just read:

a.   Select the highest quality, most natural, organic, whole foods you can get.

b.   Minimize the amount and type of food preparation used, with 50% of your food being eaten in a raw state, especially vegetables and fruits.

c.   Add a good measure of natural, gentle exercise, about 20 - 30 minutes daily.

d.   Drink at least 6 - 8 glasses of water daily, as well as your other beverages.

e.   Incorporate a specific time daily (at least 15 minutes) for deep breathing practices, and rest and relaxation.

f.   Work on developing and maintaining a healthy, optimistic, *loving* attitude, towards yourself, as well as others and the world around you.

In time you will move through your life with Ease, Confidence, Peace of Mind and Health.

What Not to Look for in This Book

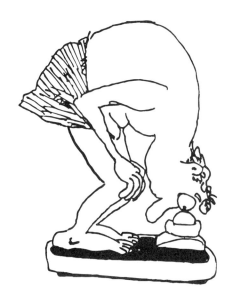

What you will not find in this book are a lot of numbers relating to the calorie counts in the foods and recipes, the sodium levels, the amount of available fiber, the level of sugar, or the number of fat grams provided. The reason is simple!

If you are eating according to the recommendations outlined throughout this book, especially those listed under **Rules for the Road,** you will never need to be concerned about how much of the potentially harmful items you are consuming.

It is the canned and packaged, processed and frozen, convenience foods, which have been prepared with large amounts of hydrogenated fats, increased levels of salt, MSG (monosodium glutamate) and simple sugars, as well as white refined flours. These white flours, regardless of the grain of origin, are devoid of the fiber found in the husk of the grain, the part removed during the milling process.

Natural foods, organically grown, and as fresh as you can find them, are nutritionally in tact, with both soluble and insoluble fibers, enzymes, natural oils in minimal amounts, low sodium levels, and naturally occurring sugars, in a more balanced and nutritionally sound base of the *vitamins, minerals and phytochemicals* so necessary for all of the biochemical and metabolic functions of a healthy body!

The preparation processes used in the menus and recipes are as simple as possible, and as minimal as possible, in order to preserve the greatest amount of the original nutritional value of the foods!

So throw away the calculator, calorie charts and fat gram books! Start simplifying your life NOW! Most importantly --- it's a new adventure, so HAVE FUN!

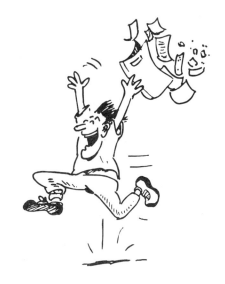

Slash the Fat

Instead of:

Bologna, Salami, Hog Dog

Bread Stuffing From Mix

Butter, Margarine (as a spread)

Butter, Margarine, Oils, Lard (in cooking)

Cream

Cream Cheese

4% Creamed Cottage Cheese

Cream Sauces for Pasta

Use:

- Sliced turkey breast
- Sliced chicken breast
- Marinated tofu slices
- Marinated and baked pork tenderloin
- Spicy tempeh slices

- Brown rice with seasoning
- Bulgur, Couscous or Oatmeal with seasoning

- Fruit preserves
- All natural sprays
- Butter sprinkles

- Nonstick pan
- Nonstick vegetable spray
- Vegetable broth
- Virgin olive oil, Canola, Sesame Oil (sparingly)

- Skim milk
- Evaporated skim milk
- 1% Lowfat milk

- Blended nonfat cottage cheese
- Lowfat cream cheese
- Lowfat ricotta
- Blended lowfat ricotta and nonfat yogurt

- Nonfat cottage cheese
- 1% lowfat cottage cheese
- Lowfat ricotta cheese

- Marinara, clam or tomato sauce w/no meat
- Blended nonfat yogurt, lemon, garlic & Parmesan

Instead of:

Use:

Cheese, hard or semi-soft

- Lowfat cheese
- Nonfat cheese
- Part-skim mozzarella or ricotta
- Lowfat soy cheese

Chili Con Carne

- Chili with ground turkey breast
- Vegetarian chili

**Cold Cereals, commercial
(flakes, puffs, crisps)**

- Grapenuts, All-Bran
- Shredded wheat, regular and spoon-size
- Wheatabix

Crackers, high-fat

- Crackers, nonfat or lowfat
- Brown rice cakes
- Wholewheat matzo crackers

Croissants, Doughnuts, Danish

- Lowfat wholegrain muffins
- Wholegrain bagel and lowfat cream cheese
- Wholegrain English muffin, rolls

Egg noodles

- Brown rice or wholegrain pasta

Fried Chicken

- Baked or grilled chicken breast, no skin
- Sauteed chicken breast nuggets, in broth

Fried Fish

- Grilled, baked or broiled finfish
- Salmon, canned in water
- Tuna, canned in water
- Broiled or boiled shellfish, occasionally

Granola Cereal

- No added fat granola
- No added fat meusli
- Any cooked grains or grain combinations

Instead of:

Hamburger, beef

Ice Cream

Margarine, Oil (in baking)

Mayonnaise

Milk Shakes, Eggnogs, Floats

Peanut Butter, Nut Butters

Pizza, Cheese and Pepperoni

Popcorn, buttered

Scalloped Potatoes, French Fries

Use:

- Turkey burger, ground breast meat
- Salmon burger
- Lowfat soy or vegetable burger

- Frozen fruit or frozen fruit bars
- Nonfat frozen yogurt (occasionally)
- Blended frozen fruit and nonfat yogurt

- Use only 1/3 to 1/2 the amount
- Applesauce
- Pureed Prunes

- Nonfat or lowfat mayonnaise
- Plain nonfat yogurt with herbs
- Nayonnaise
- Blended nonfat cottage cheese and yogurt

- Fruit nectars, whole fruit juices
- Fresh fruit frappe
- Nonfat milk or soymilk health shake

- Blended legumes with lemon and garlic
- Marinated tofu slices
- Blended soft tofu

- Vegetarian pizza on wholewheat crust

- Air-popped popcorn w/butter sprinkles
- Air-popped popcorn w/all natural sprays
- Low sodium pretzels

- Baked potatoes with nonfat yogurt topping
- Seasoned oven-baked potato wedges
- Baked sweet potatoes with nonfat yogurt

Instead of:

Use:

Sour Cream

- Plain nonfat yogurt
- Blended nonfat cottage cheese & lemon juice
- Blended lowfat ricotta and lemon juice
- Blended lowfat buttermilk & lowfat ricotta

Tortilla Chips, regular

- Baked tortilla, or baked potato, chips
- Raw vegetables

Vegetables in Butter or Cream Sauces

- Steamed fresh vegetables with butter sprinkles
- Vegetables w/lemon or lime juice, or vinegar
- Vegetables w/yogurt or buttermilk dressing
- Vegetables w/homemade nonfat dressing
- Vegetables w/Bragg's Liquid Aminos
- Vegetables w/sprinkling of Parmesan, Romano

Whipped Cream

- Whipped evaporated skim milk

Whole Eggs

- Egg whites only
- 2 to 1 whites to yolks
- 3 ounces tofu and 1 large egg

Whole Milk

- Skim milk
- 1% lowfat milk
- Evaporated skim milk

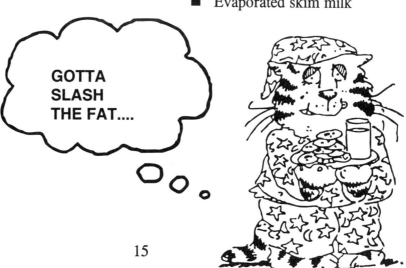

GOTTA SLASH THE FAT....

Foods to Avoid at Any Cost!

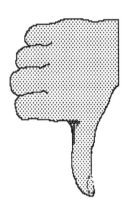

- Bacon
- Baked goods, commercial
- Butter
- Buttery crackers
- Cheeseburger, beef
- Chocolate

- Cream cheese
- Doughnuts
- Eggnog
- Fat on meats
- Fettucini Alfredo, regular
- French fries
- Fried, battered chicken, fish and meats
- Hot dog
- Ice cream, commercial
- Lard
- Luncheon meats
- Margarine

- Mayonnaise, regular
- Miracle Whip
- Oils (except olive, canola, sesame, flaxseed)
- Organ meats
- Pastries
- Peanut butter
- Potato chips, regular
- Regular cheeses
- Salad Dressings, commercial
- Sausage
- Skin on chicken, turkey and fish
- Whole milk products
- Anything fried

Let's Drink to Our Health!

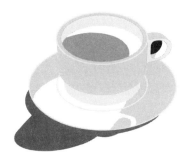

Probably one of the most common questions I get asked by my clients and patients is *"What can I drink?"* Of course this question makes sense when you look at what most people drink every day without a thought towards its detriments or benefits to their health.

What are the usual fluids included in the average diet? Here's the list:

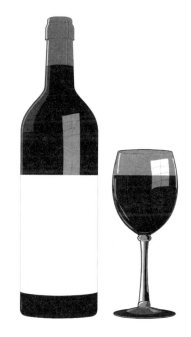

- regular coffee
- regular decaf coffee
- specialty coffees
- coke cola, regular and diet
- pepsi, regular and diet
- flavored sodas, regular and diet
- hot chocolate
- ovaltine, flavored
- black teas
- wine
- beer
- distilled liquors
- fruit flavored beverages
- reconstituted fruit juices
- fruit juices, regular and sweetened
- instant chicken or beef broth, packages or cubes

Does this look like your daily selection of beverages? Well these are the ones I am going to recommend that you either *eliminate, avoid, or drastically reduce!*

Are you now asking the question, *"What's wrong with these drinks?"* And, after all, haven't you been told that fruit juices are a healthy substitute for caffeine-based drinks? And that diet sodas are a great alternative for the diabetic, or the dieter?

Well let's take a good look at these commonly consumed beverages for a moment!

Caffeine, found in coffee, even decaffeinated coffee, cocoa, chocolate, regular black teas, cola drinks, other carbonated beverages, and many over-the-counter and prescription medications, has been associated in much of the scientific literature with most of the degenerative illnesses we know today. Even the chemicals used in the processing of the coffee beans may prove to be harmful to our health.

Sugar is found in very large amounts in most regular sodas. As there is absolutely no nutritional value in basic white sugar other than calories, loading up with all of sugar's empty calories, results generally, in a major deficit of the more nutrient-dense calories from wholesome foods.

If the aim is to provide only those foods which will do the most to enhance the health of our body, then there is no room in the diet for foods which not only, do not benefit the body, but may also have serious negative implications to our overall health!

The same is true of ***alcoholic beverages***. They are high in calories, and provide no nutritional support in the development and maintenance of health. Also, note that *all alcoholic beverages carry a warning about potential health problems*; and this statement is backed by the results of a tremendous amount of research.

Sulfites, which are used extensively in the preservation of wines, in North America, may have adverse side effects on those with allergies to this substance. Natural wines, prepared and aged properly, do not require preservatives!

Fruit juices *are often listed as a substitute for fresh fruit. Logically, how can that be?* Fresh fruit has a skin on it which contains fiber and carries many nutrients right under its surface. That skin certainly does not make it into the juice! Nor does the juice contain any of the fiber or the non-water soluble micronutrients of the flesh of the original fruit. *So again we get calories without benefits*!

There is a trend amongst people watching their weights, or limiting their sugar or caffeine intake, to substitute beverages high in these ingredients, with chicken or beef broth. Whether from a can, package, or bouillon cube, **Read the Label!** Generally these broths are loaded with **salt and MSG (monosodiumglutimate)**. The fact that a large percentage of the population has a negative reaction to MSG, anything from a dull roar of a headache to actual convulsions, negates any of its flavor-enhancing qualities.

Sodium is also used in the carbonation of most soft drinks and sodas. Most people are very aware of the sugar content in these drinks, but express great surprise about the high sodium level. Again, **Read the Label!**

Salt, or sodium, is in the news regularly, in relationship to high blood pressure, strokes, cardiovascular disease, and in general, most of the degenerative illnesses. However, if you follow the recommendations in **5 Minutes to Health**, this should not be an issue for you!

Artificially sweetened drinks and products are not recommended. Researchers are continually finding more scientific evidence to support the belief that the sweeteners being used today may have potentially harmful, long term effects, such as the development of carcinogens in our bodies.

So, to sum up the negative components of our overall drinking habits in North America, and perhaps universally, *we consume far too much caffeine, sugar, salt, MSG, artificial sweeteners and the chemicals added for preservation and shelf-life.* And unfortunately most of what we drink, apart from providing a lot of empty calories with potentially harmful side effects, does not contribute any fiber, and at most, only minimal health-giving nutrients!

As I stated at the beginning of this book, this is a **How-To** manual, **not a Why** manual. Because of the particular focus of **5 Minutes to Health**, I have just *briefly* touched on a few of the many reasons why you should avoid the above beverages. There are many books available with a detailed focus on the why's. You will find some of these listed in the resource section of this book.

Now, let's look at the abundant variety of healthy, potentially beneficial, and delicious beverages available in the marketplace. There is absolutely no reason to feel deprived! Take a look:

- pure, filtered water

- mineral water

- sparkling waters, low sodium

- spring water, low sodium

- Club Soda, low sodium

- Crystal Light drinks

- Crystal Geyser drinks

- Sundance Sparklers, low sodium

- organic fruit nectars, eg. peach, pear, apricot, etc. (has more pulp and fiber, and the micronutrients clinging to the fibers, than regular juices)

- organic apple cider

- herbal teas, leaves or bags, eg. those by Good Earth, Celestial Seasonings, Great Eastern Sun (Japanese organic Kukicha teas). **Read the Label!** Herbal teas are **not black teas with fruit or flower flavorings added!** Many large, commercial companies have this type of flavored tea available. *Avoid in the name of your health!*

- herbal teas for therapeutic purposes, eg. constipation, runny nose, nausea, etc., produced by companies such as Traditional Medicinals and Herba-Fed.

- iced herbal teas, made either with regular brewed tea, chilled and iced, or with the new teas which can be brewed in cold water, eg. those by Celestial Seasonings.

- Chinese green tea, from China

- ginger tea, made with the natural root, or tea bags (see recipe)

- rosehip tea, leaves or bags

- red clover tea, leaves

- nettle tea, leaves

- mint tea/peppermint tea, leaves or bags

- alfalfa tea, leaves or bags

- ginseng tea, made with the natural root, or tea bags

- V-8 juice, low sodium

- tomato juice, low sodium

- organic coffee beans, use sparingly

- organic decaffeinated coffee beans, use sparingly

- postum, a grain-based coffee alternative; can also make postum latte, by using heated soymilk, low-fat acidophilus milk, or regular nonfat milk.

- Cafix, a grain-based coffee substitute; can also make Cafix latte by using heated soymilk, low-fat acidophilus milk, or regular nonfat milk.

- Take-5 Vegetable Refresher powder by Custom Foods Inc., a healthy tingling vegetable and citrus based drink; delicious hot or cold.

- Super Green Pro-96, by Nature' Life, a natural high protein, nutrient-loaded powder that can be used alone in water or soymilk, or in health drinks.

Note: *Have fun with your beverages!*

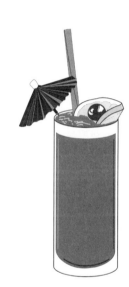

- Mix different varieties of herbal teas to create your own flavors of hot or iced teas.

- Club soda or mineral water can be added to fruit nectars.

- A Virgin Mary can be made by spicing up tomato juice or V-8 juice.

- Sparkling beverages can be added to iced tea to perk it up with the bubbles.

- If you drink a little wine or beer, look for naturally prepared, without added sulfites.

Snack Attack!

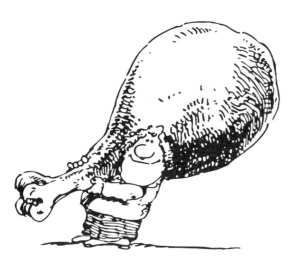

So you've got the munchies! And they're fierce! You're craving something -- *anything* -- to take the edge off! And all that you can think of, at this moment, are the foods I have recommended for you to avoid. After all, isn't that what we mean when we think of snack foods? *Aren't they the forbidden delights?* Those foods loaded with fats, sugars, salt and cholesterol?
WRONG!

In light of the fact that most of us can't think straight when we're in the middle of a snack attack, I felt that it was only fair to provide a ready list of delicious alternatives to the regular, much advertised variety of *"junk foods"* which are so available, and so eye-catchingly displayed, in the most obvious sections of your local grocery or convenience stores.

The following list is by no means the last word on snack foods!

But it is a very good base from which to start when you can't move your thoughts past potato chips and sour cream dips, or pizza loaded with cheese and pepperoni, or a box of chocolate chip cookies, or a pint of Hagen Das ice cream.

And remember, that apart from all of the suggestions outlined here, *we all have leftovers from time to time that can be eaten* as they are, or can be incorporated into other dishes, for tasty alternatives to the typical convenience snack foods available in every corner store in America. **Just think low fat, low sugar, low sodium, low cholesterol and high fiber!** And then make your wise choices accordingly.

In the References and Resources section of this book, you will

find listed some of the companies that produce healthy alternatives to the usual high fat, sodium-laden, heavily sugared, and cholesterol-loaded foods and condiments. Many of these products are available in your local supermarket, or health food store. If you can't find the products anywhere, write to, or call the company, for information on how and where to get them. Several companies actually have mail order services set up, so that no matter where you live, or how remote the area is, they will ship their products to you.

Now on to the list of snack ideas. Here's to snack attacks !

Remember, this is a new adventure. Have fun with it! Copy this list and put it somewhere obvious so you can refer to it before you uncontrollably crunch and munch!

- 1/2 wholegrain bagel with fruit preserves
- 1/2 wholegrain bagel with blended lowfat ricotta cheese and fruit preserves
- air-popped popcorn, sprayed with all natural flavor sprays
- air-popped popcorn, seasoned with herbs
- air-popped popcorn, seasoned with garlic-flavored butter sprinkles
- apple slices with tofu cheese sticks
- apple slices
- applesauce and plain, nonfat yogurt
- baked potato topped with nonfat refried beans and nonfat grated cheese
- baked potato topped with salsa or Dijon mustard
- baked potato topped with nonfat yogurt seasoned with herbs
- baked potato chips and seasoned nonfat yogurt dip, or salsa, or the combination
- baked tortilla chips with salsa
- bean burrito with corn tortilla and nonfat refried beans
- blended frozen banana
- broiled nonfat grated cheese and sliced tomato on wholegrain toast
- brown rice, heated, and served with Bragg's Liquid Aminos
- brown rice, heated, and served with seasoned nonfat yogurt
- brown rice, leftover, with vanilla soymilk, fresh fruit, and a teaspoon pure maple syrup
- buckwheat, heated, and served with seasoned nonfat yogurt
- celery with curried nonfat cream cheese and chives
- cup-a-soup, or meal-in-a-cup, dehydrated, lowfat, low sodium varieties
- fresh fruit, nonfat plain yogurt and cinnamon whipped together
- frozen grapes or frozen chunks of mango, pineapple or papaya
- fruit frappe, with blended fresh fruit and ice cubes
- fruit nectar popsicles
- fruit, pureed and frozen in ice cube trays
- fruit slices with nonfat yogurt dip, flavored with almond extract and pure maple syrup

- garlic wholewheat sourdough toast using all natural flavor sprays
- leftover pasta and vegetables mixed together as a salad with nonfat dressing
- leftover steamed vegetables with seasoned nonfat yogurt
- low sodium pretzels
- marinated tofu slices on wholegrain bread or roll
- milkshake of nonfat milk or soymilk and frozen fruit
- millet, heated, and served with Bragg's Liquid Aminos
- miso soup with tofu cubes and sliced green onions
- mulled organic apple cider
- no added fat granola and soymilk
- nonfat cheese and nonfat wholegrain crackers
- nonfat frozen yogurt (use sparingly)
- nonfat, fruit juice-sweetened, cookies
- nonfat granola bar
- nonfat or lowfat wholegrain or bran muffins
- nonfat wholegrain crackers and nonfat cottage or ricotta cheese
- nonfat, wholewheat, wholegrain or rye crackers
- organic green salad with nonfat dressing
- plain, nonfat yogurt with fresh fruit
- potato salad with seasoned, nonfat yogurt or buttermilk dressing
- raw vegetable strips (e.g., carrots, celery, broccoli, turnip, cauliflower, mushrooms, green and red peppers, cucumber, zucchini) with yogurt dip
- raw vegetable strips and salsa
- raw vegetables with nonfat refried beans
- rye crisps or rice cakes spread with lowfat cream cheese (use sparingly)
- seasoned baked potato wedges
- seasoned blended chickpeas with wholewheat pita wedges
- soycheese and nonfat wholegrain crackers
- vanilla soymilk
- wholegrain breadsticks
- wholegrain English muffin pizza, using grated nonfat cheese and tomato sauce
- wholegrain graham crackers
- wholegrain toast with apple butter
- wholewheat toast with blended applesauce and nonfat cottage cheese

Help for Indigestion

Whether healthy or ill, we all at times, due to lack of rest, overwork, or undue stress, experience that uncomfortable feeling of indigestion with the accompanying gas, after we've eaten a meal. This seems to increase as we get older, possibly due to a decrease over the years, in the amount of enzymes produced by our bodies. The problem definitely appears to be much more pronounced in someone dealing with a chronic illness, especially of the degenerative nature, such as cancer, A.I.D.S., heart disease, diabetes, etc. However there are several steps that can be taken to alleviate the problem.

1. **Eat only until you feel satisfied.** Beyond that puts added stress on your overworked body to digest and distribute or store the extra that it does not need at that time.

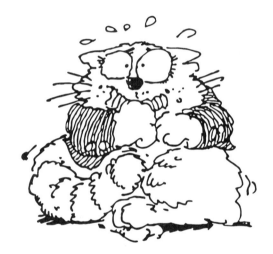

2. **Avoid eating when you feel anxious, uptight, worried or overly stressed.** Take the time to calm yourself, prior to eating, by using techniques such as deep breathing, yoga, relaxing music, or an unhurried bath with only the light of candles.

3. **Eat your larger meals earlier in the day, making the evening meal your lightest meal of the day.** This way the body gets the greater intake of food when it is less tired from the day's activities and therefore, most able to handle digestion.

4. **Changing the way you combine your foods at a meal may have an impact** on the way your body handles the intake. Because of different rates of digestion, some foods which are digested more quickly, such as fruits, do not mix well with more slowly digested foods, such as meats. This has made a big difference for many of my clients! *Here are some general guidelines:*

Bad Combinations:

- Starches with meat, fish, poultry, nuts, seeds, soybeans
- Any fruit with a starch
- Any fruit with a protein, e.g., meat, fish, poultry, nuts, seeds, soybeans
- Any fruits, except tomatoes, with any vegetables
- Acid fruits (citrus, pineapple) with sweet fruits (dried fruits, banana)
- Oils (vegetable oils, butter, margarine) with starches
- Melons (any variety) with any other foods
- More than 4 vegetables at a meal
- More than 3 fruits at a meal
- More than 1 protein food at a meal
- More than 1 starchy food at a meal

Good Combinations:

- Leafy greens with meat, fish, poultry, nuts, seeds, soybeans
- Vegetables with starches
- Grains with all legumes except soybeans
- 3 starchy vegetables (maximum), e.g., potatoes, squash, at a meal
- Leafy greens with oils
- Acid fruits (citrus, pineapple) with oils
- Subacid fruits (e.g., apple, pear, grapes, mango, papaya, etc.) with oils

(See the *Resources Section* for recommendations on books, materials, and organizations which may be able to assist you.)

5. Grated raw daikon radish, eaten as a relish with a meal, has been used for centuries in the Orient, as a digestive aid. In it's raw state it is loaded with enzymes!

6. Fresh ginger, grated into salad dishes, or added to cooked dishes, not only adds a delicious flavor, but appears to stimulate more efficient digestion of the foods it is eaten with. *Ginger tea,* either hot or iced, (see recipe) is an excellent accompaniment to a meal.

7. **Fresh, natural, nonfat yogurt which contains live cultures,** including *lactobacillus acidophilus and bifidus cultures,* as well as *lactobacillus bulgaricus and streptococcus thermophilus yogurt cultures,* creates a healthy environment in the colon, by killing unhealthy bacteria. *Yogurt, acidophilus milk, and kefir in the plain, nonfat form,* facilitate digestion and increase resistance to infections. *Yogurt's active bacteria, and by-products of the bacteria's activity,* in the digestive tract and colon, have been reported to boost the immune system, to serve as natural antibiotics against infection, and to act as suppressants of the activity in the colon that converts harmless bacteria into carcinogens.

8. **Lactose intolerance, due to a deficiency of lactase, a digestive enzyme, which digests lactose,** the milk sugar in milk and dairy products, can result in gas when the undigested milk sugar, reaches the colon. *Yogurt does not generally create a problem* for lactase deficient individuals. The active bacteria used in the preparation of yogurt, breaks down the lactose in the process.

9. **A sudden switch to high fiber foods,** especially wholegrains and legumes, as well as an increase in raw vegetables and fruits, can result in the production of gas. Generally, this will lessen and return to normal after a few weeks. *One strategy would be to implement a gradual increase in fiber intake,* to allow the colon time to adjust.

10. **Swallowing air can create a severe gas problem.** This occurs while eating, drinking, chewing gum, smoking, belching or breathing deeply and rapidly with your mouth open, as during physical activity. *Take smaller bites of food, chew food slowly with your mouth closed, and <u>drink</u> liquids, not gulp liquids, before or after meals, not during meals.*

11. Foods which seem to create a problem in their whole form, may be more digestible in a more broken down, more bioavailable form:

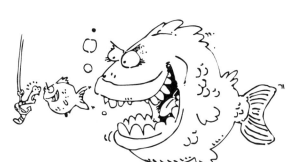

a.   ground up beans in hummus or nonfat refried beans

b.   blenderized vegetables, used in sauces or smooth soups

c.   blenderized fruits in healthy protein drinks and frappes

d.   any of the above, blended with yogurt, acidophilus milk, buttermilk, kefir, or the live acidophilus culture itself

e.   the addition of fresh ginger root or fresh daikon radish to any of the above blended products may assist digestion and prevent gas

12. The use of enzyme supplements about 15 minutes prior to eating a meal may ease or eliminate the problem. Start with a ***basic papaya and pineapple enzyme supplement***, available in most health food stores, or ***Beano***, available in most pharmacies, and many grocery stores. Seek the advice of a qualified health professional, eg. a Registered Dietitian or a Medical Doctor, should the problem continue.

13. Drink adequate fluids daily. At least 6 to 8, 8 ounce glasses every day! *Water is essential for every process or function within the body! Including Digestion.*

14. Specific, basic yoga exercises can significantly alleviate the production of gas, or quicken its release from the body. See the **Resources** section for recommendations on magazines and organizations which may be able to assist you. Also listed is a good contact for audio and videotapes: The Motivational Tape Company.

A Word About Supplements

As this is a book focused on food and healthy eating, I do not plan to devote much space to a discussion on supplements. However, because the question of whether or not to incorporate their use into a healthy nutritionally fit program always comes up, along with the question of, if so, what and how much, it is apparently an important enough issue to at least provide a few basic guidelines.

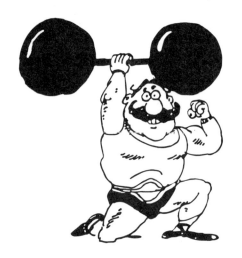

The truth is that everyone's body is different, with varying requirements for each of the multitude of nutrients. And when an individual follows a dietary regime which is predominantly made up of living foods, such as wholegrains, fresh fruits and vegetables and cultured foods, eg. tempeh, miso and yogurt, not only are most, if not all, of their needs met, but the body becomes so tuned into its needs that it signals deficiencies through cravings for certain healthy foods, or reacts negatively to the intake of others. To determine the specific requirements of an individual, the services of a qualified health professional, such as a Registered Dietitian, an M.D. who specializes in nutrition, or a related health practitioner with a background in biochemistry and human nutrition, and perhaps a strong working knowledge of herbs, should be employed.

In my practice, I believe that it is often necessary to incorporate some additional supplemental therapy. Therefore, I regularly recommend a variety of basic supplements, along with the fairly radical shift in nutritional intake outlined in this book. Some reasons for implementing such guidelines are as follows:

1.   Almost everyone I see in my own practice has been on a nutritionally deficient dietary regime for years prior to our work together.

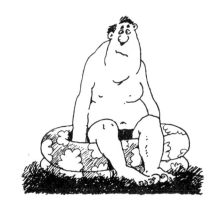

2.   Their is a need for a reduced caloric intake below the recommended level for optimum nutritional support, in order to reduce and balance the individual's weight.

3.   The client has just been diagnosed with moderate to severe symptoms of a degenerative illness, such as heart disease, stroke, cancer, diabetes, chronic fatigue syndrome, arthritis, or AIDS.

4.   Any combination of the above listed factors.

I will stress here, however, that under no circumstances should nutritional supplements replace a balanced intake of healthy, wholesome, and simply prepared foods. The word **supplement** means just that, a "desirable addition" (as defined by Webster's dictionary) to whatever else you are including. Supplement does not mean, on its own! *It is to be taken with something.*

Furthermore, supplements are made up of micronutrients, including vitamins, minerals, and phytochemicals, which are so small they can only be seen by the eye under a microscope. These tiny molecules require macronutrients, the proteins, carbohydrates and fats in our foods, which are visible to the eye, to carry them throughout the body to the places where they are needed. In other words, they are carried to the body's many cellular factories, for breakdown into even more microscopic molecules, to be used for the millions of bodily metabolic processes.

So you see, **if you wake up and swallow a handful of supplements with a cup of coffee every morning, you are as good as flushing those nutrients down the toilet!** They have nothing to work with. I cannot begin to count the number of clients who, after only one month of incorporating this change into their morning regime, i.e. taking their supplements with food instead of on an empty stomach, report increased energy and a greater sense of well-being! Why not try it and see for yourself?

As far as what supplements to take, I recommend a good basic, and preferably natural (for increased bioavailability), vitamin and mineral supplement to start. The best varieties are those which provide from approximately 100 to 300% of the USRDA (Recommended Daily Allowances). With so much scientific research and information supporting the need for antioxidants and phytochemicals (plant chemicals), I usually encourage the addition of a good natural antioxidant combination as well. And based on the massive amount of scientific data expounding the wide range of benefits provided by Vitamin C, from protection against environmental pollutants and preservatives in food, to assisting the body in wounding healing and handling stress, I recommend an additional intake of 2000 to 4000 milligrams of buffered Vitamin C, depending on my client's present nutrition and lifestyle habits, body weight and techniques for handling day to day stress.

For supplements, as with diet, quality, not quantity, is the principle!

Shop For Health
Stocking the Refrigerator and Pantry with Healthy Choices

The Pyramid of Power which follows, is based on the USDA's Food Guide Pyramid. However, the Pyramid you will explore in **this** book is power-packed with only the most natural, most unprocessed foods available today! At most, the foods listed, contain only minimal amounts of added fats, sugars, sodium, caffeine, preservatives, food colorings, or cholesterol. If you select your foods from this chart, you will have no problem achieving optimum health with boundless energy.

To assist you with the *shop* and *stock* process, you will find, following the Pyramid, a comprehensive shopping list, which is broken down into the food groups from the Pyramid, plus sections for **Condiments and Flavorings,** for **Dried Herbs, Spices and Vegetable Seasonings,** for **Beverages,** and for **Miscellaneous Items.**

Remember that this is an *extensive list*, demonstrating the incredible variety of foods, beverages and seasonings available for the development and maintenance of your health! By no means do you have to immediately run out and buy everything listed on your first shopping trip. Start by purchasing the items you are most familiar with, or that appeal to you most. Then over time, experiment with the items listed that you have never tried before. You will find ideas, suggestions and recipes throughout this book for ways to use the various foods listed.

The most fun will be enjoyed by those who view this wholesome, natural way of shopping and eating as an exciting new adventure!

With respect to the multitude of fresh fruits and vegetables available, as much as possible *buy them in season*. This varies according to the area in which you live. If you are unsure about the seasonal breakdown where you live, you can contact the Department of Agriculture and they will send this information out to you. Your local library may also be able to provide you with further information, or resources for information, on this matter.

Avoid the myriad of canned fruits and vegetables throughout the vast expanse of the grocery store shelves. Apart from the high salt or sugar solutions saturating the products sitting in those cans, the amount of heat and handling involved in the canning process of those fruits and vegetables, has virtually destroyed most of the nutrient value and all of the active enzymes, resulting in a much less than satisfactory texture, taste and nutritional component. *Believe me, once you readjust your taste buds to the taste, texture and aroma of fresh produce, you will never open another can.*

The few canned or bottled products included in the following lists are those which are changed very little in the processing, in comparison to the preparation at home, which may be lengthy and/or time-consuming. *Choose bottles over cans whenever possible!*

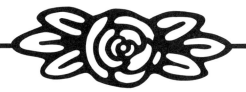

ntil one is committed there is hesitancy, the chance to draw back, always ineffectiveness. Concerning all acts of initiative (and Creation), there is one elementary truth, the ignorance of which kills countless ideas and splendid plans: that the moment one definitely commits oneself, then providence moves too. All sorts of things occur to help one that would otherwise never have occurred. A whole stream of events issues from the decision, raising in one's favor all manner of unforeseen incidents and meetings and material assistance, which no man could have dreamt would have come his way. I have learned a deep respect for one of Goethe's couplets:

Whatever you can do, or dream you can, begin it.
Boldness has genius, power and magic in it.

-- Goethe

W.N. Murray

Pyramid of Power

FATS, OILS AND SWEETS
Use Sparingly

Sucanat
Canola Oil
Nayonnaise
Pure Honey
Fruit Preserves
Fresh Avocados
Romano Cheese
Olives (sparingly)
Pure Maple Syrup
Parmesan Cheese
Pure Virgin Olive Oil
Organic Coffee Beans
Nonfat Salad Dressing
Lowfat Salad Dressing
Butter-Olive Oil Spread
Cold Pressed Sesame Oil
Cold Pressed Flaxseed Oil

Almonds
Almond Butter
Sesame Seeds
Sunflower Seeds
Tofu
Tempeh
Miso
Turkey, Free Range
Ground Turkey Breast
Chicken, Free Range
Eggs, Free Range
Venison
Buffalo Meat
Fish, Free Range
Fish, Deep Water
Canned Sardines
Canned Tuna in Water
Canned Salmon in Water
Shellfish
Rabbit
Pork Tenderloin
Imitation Crabmeat (Pollock Fish)
Dried Beans, Peas & Lentils
Canned Beans, Peas & Lentils
Canned Chick Peas
Nonfat Refried Beans
Canned Vegetarian Chili
Lima Beans
Tahini (Sesame Seed Butter)

Nonfat Yogurt
Nonfat Kefir
Lowfat Acidophilus Milk
Nonfat Cottage Cheese
Reduced Fat Ricotta Cheese
Mozarella, Part Skim
Reduced/Nonfat Cheeses
Lowfat Cream Cheese
Soymilk, Plain & Flavored
Lowfat Buttermilk
Nonfat & 1% Skim Milk
Evaporated Skim Milk
Soy Cheeses
Rice Dream Milk

MILK, YOGURT &
CHEESE GROUP
2 - 3 Servings

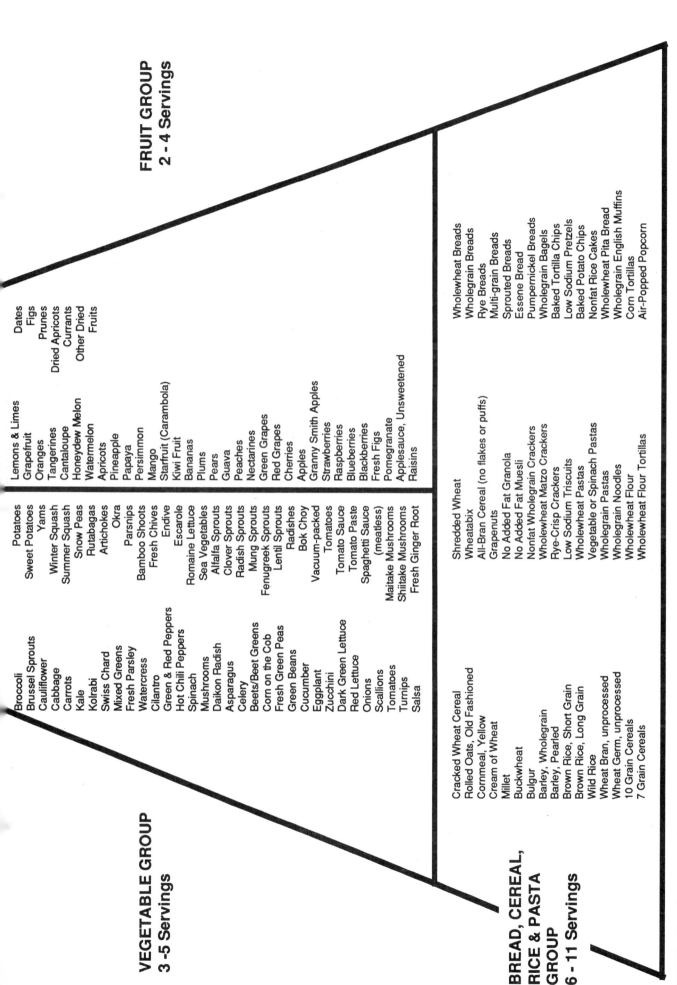

FRUIT GROUP
2 - 4 Servings

Lemons & Limes
Grapefruit
Oranges
Tangerines
Cantaloupe
Honeydew Melon
Watermelon
Apricots
Pineapple
Papaya
Persimmon
Mango
Starfruit (Carambola)
Kiwi Fruit
Bananas
Plums
Pears
Guava
Peaches
Nectarines
Green Grapes
Red Grapes
Cherries
Apples
Granny Smith Apples
Strawberries
Raspberries
Blueberries
Blackberries
Fresh Figs
Pomegranate
Applesauce, Unsweetened
Raisins

Dates
Figs
Prunes
Dried Apricots
Currants
Other Dried Fruits

VEGETABLE GROUP
3 -5 Servings

Broccoli
Brussel Sprouts
Cauliflower
Cabbage
Carrots
Kale
Kolrabi
Swiss Chard
Mixed Greens
Fresh Parsley
Watercress
Cilantro
Green & Red Peppers
Hot Chili Peppers
Spinach
Mushrooms
Daikon Radish
Asparagus
Celery
Beets/Beet Greens
Corn on the Cob
Fresh Green Peas
Green Beans
Cucumber
Eggplant
Zucchini
Dark Green Lettuce
Red Lettuce
Onions
Scallions
Tomatoes
Turnips
Salsa

Potatoes
Sweet Potatoes
Yams
Winter Squash
Summer Squash
Snow Peas
Rutabagas
Artichokes
Okra
Parsnips
Bamboo Shoots
Fresh Chives
Endive
Escarole
Romaine Lettuce
Sea Vegetables
Alfalfa Sprouts
Clover Sprouts
Radish Sprouts
Mung Sprouts
Fenugreek Sprouts
Lentil Sprouts
Radishes
Bok Choy
Vacuum-packed Tomatoes
Tomato Sauce
Tomato Paste
Spaghetti Sauce (meatless)
Maitake Mushrooms
Shiitake Mushrooms
Fresh Ginger Root

BREAD, CEREAL,
RICE & PASTA
GROUP
6 - 11 Servings

Cracked Wheat Cereal
Rolled Oats, Old Fashioned
Cornmeal, Yellow
Cream of Wheat
Millet
Buckwheat
Bulgur
Barley, Wholegrain
Barley, Pearled
Brown Rice, Short Grain
Brown Rice, Long Grain
Wild Rice
Wheat Bran, unprocessed
Wheat Germ, unprocessed
10 Grain Cereals
7 Grain Cereals

Shredded Wheat
Wheatabix
All-Bran Cereal (no flakes or puffs)
Grapenuts
No Added Fat Granola
No Added Fat Muesli
Nonfat Wholegrain Crackers
Wholewheat Matzo Crackers
Rye-Crisp Crackers
Low Sodium Triscuits
Wholewheat Pastas
Vegetable or Spinach Pastas
Wholegrain Pastas
Wholegrain Noodles
Wholewheat Flour
Wholewheat Flour Tortillas

Wholewheat Breads
Wholegrain Breads
Rye Breads
Multi-grain Breads
Sprouted Breads
Essene Bread
Pumpernickel Breads
Wholegrain Bagels
Baked Tortilla Chips
Low Sodium Pretzels
Baked Potato Chips
Nonfat Rice Cakes
Wholewheat Pita Bread
Wholegrain English Muffins
Corn Tortillas
Air-Popped Popcorn

NOTE: For best results using this Pyramid, begin by selecting more foods from the lower layers of the multi-layered chart, with portion sizes of food items decreasing as you climb to the top of the Pyramid.

5 Minutes to Health Shopping List

Bread, Cereal, Rice & Pasta:

- ☐ 7 & 10 Grain Cereals
- ☐ Air-Popped Popcorn
- ☐ All-Bran Cereal (no flakes or puffs)
- ☐ Bagels, Wholegrain
- ☐ Barley, Wholegrain & Pearled
- ☐ Breads, Rye, Pumpernickel
- ☐ Breads, Sprouted & Multi-grain
- ☐ Breads, Whole Wheat & Wholegrain
- ☐ Brown Rice, Short & Long Grain
- ☐ Buckwheat
- ☐ Bulgur
- ☐ Cornmeal, Yellow
- ☐ Cracked Wheat Cereal
- ☐ Crackers, Nonfat & Lowfat, Wholegrain
- ☐ Cream of Wheat
- ☐ English Muffins, Wholegrain
- ☐ Essene Bread
- ☐ Granola, No Added Fat
- ☐ Grapenuts
- ☐ Matzo Crackers, Whole Wheat
- ☐ Millet
- ☐ Muesli, No Added Fat
- ☐ Noodles, Wholegrain
- ☐ Pastas, Vegetable & Spinach
- ☐ Pastas, Whole Wheat & Whole Grain
- ☐ Pita Bread, Whole Wheat
- ☐ Potato Chips, Baked
- ☐ Pretzels, Low Sodium
- ☐ Rice Cakes, Nonfat
- ☐ Rolled Oats, Old Fashioned
- ☐ Rye-Crisp Crackers
- ☐ Shredded Wheat
- ☐ Tortilla Chips, Baked
- ☐ Tortillas, Corn
- ☐ Tortillas, Whole Wheat
- ☐ Triscuits, Low Sodium
- ☐ Wheat Bran, unprocessed
- ☐ Wheat Germ, unprocessed
- ☐ Wheatabix
- ☐ Whole Wheat Flour
- ☐ Wild Rice

Vegetable Group:

- ☐ Alfalfa Sprouts
- ☐ Artichokes
- ☐ Asparagus
- ☐ Bamboo Shoots
- ☐ Beets/Beet Greens
- ☐ Bok Choy
- ☐ Broccoli
- ☐ Brussel Sprouts
- ☐ Cabbage
- ☐ Carrots
- ☐ Cauliflower
- ☐ Celery
- ☐ Cilantro
- ☐ Clover Sprouts
- ☐ Corn on the Cob
- ☐ Cucumber
- ☐ Daikon Radish
- ☐ Dark Green Lettuce
- ☐ Eggplant
- ☐ Endive
- ☐ Escarole
- ☐ Fenugreek Sprouts
- ☐ Fresh Chives
- ☐ Fresh Ginger Root
- ☐ Fresh Green Peas
- ☐ Fresh Parsley
- ☐ Green & Red Peppers
- ☐ Green Beans
- ☐ Hot Chili Peppers
- ☐ Kale
- ☐ Kolrabi
- ☐ Lentil Sprouts
- ☐ Maitake Mushrooms
- ☐ Mixed Greens
- ☐ Mung Sprouts
- ☐ Mushrooms
- ☐ Okra
- ☐ Onions
- ☐ Parsnips
- ☐ Potatoes
- ☐ Radish Sprouts
- ☐ Radishes
- ☐ Red Lettuce
- ☐ Romaine Lettuce
- ☐ Rutabagas
- ☐ Salsa
- ☐ Scallions
- ☐ Sea Vegetables
- ☐ Shiitake Mushrooms
- ☐ Snow Peas
- ☐ Spaghetti Sauce (meatless)
- ☐ Spinach
- ☐ Summer Squash
- ☐ Sweet Potatoes
- ☐ Swiss Chard
- ☐ Tomato Paste
- ☐ Tomato Sauce
- ☐ Tomatoes
- ☐ Turnips
- ☐ Vacuum-packed Tomatoes
- ☐ Watercress
- ☐ Winter Squash
- ☐ Yams
- ☐ Zucchini

Fruits:

- ☐ Apples
- ☐ Applesauce, Unsweetened
- ☐ Apricots, Fresh/Dried
- ☐ Bananas
- ☐ Blackberries
- ☐ Blueberries
- ☐ Cantaloupe
- ☐ Cherries
- ☐ Currants
- ☐ Dates
- ☐ Dried Peaches, Apples, Bananas
- ☐ Dried Tropical Fruits
- ☐ Figs, Fresh/Dried
- ☐ Granny Smith Apples
- ☐ Grapefruit
- ☐ Green Grapes
- ☐ Guava
- ☐ Honeydew Melon
- ☐ Kiwi Fruit
- ☐ Lemons & Limes
- ☐ Mango
- ☐ Nectarines
- ☐ Oranges
- ☐ Papaya
- ☐ Peaches
- ☐ Pears
- ☐ Persimmon
- ☐ Pineapple
- ☐ Plums
- ☐ Pomegranate
- ☐ Prunes
- ☐ Raisins
- ☐ Raspberries
- ☐ Red Grapes
- ☐ Starfruit (Carambola)
- ☐ Strawberries
- ☐ Tangerines
- ☐ Watermelon

Milk, Yogurt & Cheese:

- ☐ Acidophilus Milk, Lowfat
- ☐ Buttermilk, Lowfat
- ☐ Cream Cheese, Lowfat
- ☐ Evaporated Skim Milk
- ☐ Kefir, Nonfat
- ☐ Mozarella, Part Skim
- ☐ Nonfat Cheeses, Reduced Fat & Nonfat
- ☐ Rice Dream Milk
- ☐ Ricotta Cheese, Reduced Fat
- ☐ Ricotta Cheese, Nonfat
- ☐ Skim Milk, Nonfat & 1%
- ☐ Soy Cheeses
- ☐ Soymilk, Plain & Flavored
- ☐ Yogurt, Nonfat, Plain

Poultry, Fish, Meat, Eggs, Dry Beans & Nuts:

- ☐ Ahi Tuna
- ☐ Almond Butter
- ☐ Almonds
- ☐ Buffalo Meat
- ☐ Canned Beans, Peas & Lentils
- ☐ Canned Chick Peas (Garbanzo Beans)

- ☐ Canned Salmon in Water
- ☐ Canned Sardines
- ☐ Canned Tuna in Water
- ☐ Canned Vegetarian Chili
- ☐ Chicken Breast, Free Range
- ☐ Dried Beans, Peas & Lentils
- ☐ Eggs, Free Range
- ☐ Fish, Deep Water/Free Range
- ☐ Ground Turkey Breast
- ☐ Haddock
- ☐ Halibut
- ☐ Imitation Crabmeat (Pollock Fish)
- ☐ Lima Beans
- ☐ Mackerel
- ☐ Miso
- ☐ Refried Beans, Nonfat
- ☐ Pork Tenderloin
- ☐ Rabbit
- ☐ Red Snapper
- ☐ Salmon, Fresh
- ☐ Sea Bass
- ☐ Sesame Seeds
- ☐ Shellfish
- ☐ Sunflower Seeds
- ☐ Swordfish
- ☐ Tahini (Sesame Seed Butter)
- ☐ Tempeh
- ☐ Tofu
- ☐ Turkey Breast, Free Range
- ☐ Venison

Fats, Oils & Sweets:
- ☐ Avocados, Fresh
- ☐ Butter (sparingly)
- ☐ Canola Oil
- ☐ Coffee Beans, Organic
- ☐ Flaxseed Oil, Cold Pressed
- ☐ Fruit Preserves
- ☐ Honey, Pure
- ☐ Maple Syrup, Pure
- ☐ Nayonnaise
- ☐ Olive Oil, Pure Virgin
- ☐ Olives (sparingly)
- ☐ Paramesan Cheese
- ☐ Romano Cheese
- ☐ Salad Dressings, Nonfat
- ☐ Salad Dressings, Lowfat
- ☐ Sesame Oil, Cold Pressed
- ☐ Sucanat

Condiments & Flavorings:
- ☐ Bernard Jensen's Vegetable Broth & Seasoning
- ☐ Bragg's Liquid Aminos
- ☐ Butter Buds
- ☐ Capers
- ☐ Flavor Extract, Pure Almond
- ☐ Flavor Extract, Pure Lemon
- ☐ Flavor Extract, Pure Orange
- ☐ Flavor Extract, Sherry, Brandy
- ☐ Flavor Extract, Pure Vanilla
- ☐ Flavor Sprays, Tryson House

- ☐ Gayelord Hauser's Vegetable Broth
- ☐ Hot Pepper Sauce
- ☐ Molly McButter
- ☐ Molly McButter, Garlic
- ☐ Mustard, Dijon
- ☐ Mustard, Stoneground
- ☐ Nutritional Yeast
- ☐ Seaweed, Kelp
- ☐ Seaweed, Nori
- ☐ Seaweed, Wakame
- ☐ Soy Sauce, Low Sodium
- ☐ Taco Sauce, Green
- ☐ Taco Sauce, Red
- ☐ Tamari Sauce
- ☐ Tobasco Sauce
- ☐ Vinegar, Balsamic
- ☐ Vinegar, Cider
- ☐ Vinegar, Malt
- ☐ Vinegar, Rice
- ☐ Vinegar, Wine

Dried Herbs, Spices & Vegetable Seasonings:
- ☐ Allspice, Ground & Whole
- ☐ Anise
- ☐ Basil Leaves
- ☐ Bay Leaves
- ☐ Bell Pepper Flakes, Dried
- ☐ Caraway Seeds
- ☐ Cardamom, Ground
- ☐ Cayenne Pepper
- ☐ Celery Seeds
- ☐ Chervil
- ☐ Chili Powder, Mild & Regular
- ☐ Chilis, Dried & Crushed
- ☐ Chilis, Dried & Whole
- ☐ Chives Dried
- ☐ Cilantro, Dried
- ☐ Cinnamon, Ground & Sticks
- ☐ Cloves, Ground & Whole
- ☐ Coriander
- ☐ Cumin, Ground
- ☐ Curry Powder
- ☐ Dill Seeds
- ☐ Dill Weed
- ☐ Fennel Seeds
- ☐ Fine Herbs
- ☐ Garlic Powder
- ☐ Garlic, Minced
- ☐ Ginger, Powdered
- ☐ Horseradish, Powdered/ Prepared
- ☐ Italian Seasoning
- ☐ Mace, Ground
- ☐ Marjoram
- ☐ Mint Flakes & Leaves
- ☐ Mrs. Dash/Spicy Mrs. Dash
- ☐ Mustard, Dry
- ☐ Mustard Seeds
- ☐ Nutmeg, Ground
- ☐ Onion Flakes
- ☐ Onion Powder
- ☐ Oregano Leaves
- ☐ Paprika
- ☐ Parsley, Dried

- ☐ Pepper, Black
- ☐ Pepper, Red
- ☐ Pepper, White
- ☐ Peppercorns, Black
- ☐ Poppy Seeds
- ☐ Poultry Seasoning
- ☐ Rosemary Leaves
- ☐ Rosemary, Ground
- ☐ Saffron
- ☐ Sage
- ☐ Salad Herbs
- ☐ Sesame Seeds
- ☐ Tarragon Leaves
- ☐ Thyme Leaves
- ☐ Thyme, Ground
- ☐ Turmeric
- ☐ Vegetable Flakes & Powders

Beverages:
- ☐ Cafix
- ☐ Chinese Green Tea
- ☐ Club Soda, Low Sodium
- ☐ Crystal Geyser Fruit Drinks
- ☐ Fruit Nectars, Unsweetened
- ☐ Ginger Tea, Root or Bags
- ☐ Ginseng Tea, Root or Bags
- ☐ Herbal Teas, Leaves or Bags
- ☐ Iced Herbal Teas
- ☐ Mineral Water
- ☐ Mint Tea, Leaves or Bags
- ☐ Nettle Tea, Leaves
- ☐ Organic Coffee Beans (sparingly)
- ☐ Organic Decaf Coffee Beans
- ☐ Perrier Water
- ☐ Postum
- ☐ Red Clover Tea, Leaves
- ☐ Rosehip Tea, Bags or Leaves
- ☐ Spring Water, Low Sodium
- ☐ Sundance Sparklers
- ☐ Super Green Pro-96, Nature's Life
- ☐ Take-5 Vegetable Refresher
- ☐ Tomato Juice, Low Sodium
- ☐ V-8 Juice, Low Sodium
- ☐ Water, Pure, Filtered

Miscellaneous Items:
- ☐ Baking Powder, Aluminum-free
- ☐ Baking Soda
- ☐ Blue Green Algae, e.g. Cell Tech
- ☐ Canned Soups, Health Valley
- ☐ Canned Split Pea Soup, Andersen's
- ☐ Chlorella
- ☐ Fat Free Cookies, Health Valley
- ☐ Fat Free Jammers, Auburn Farms
- ☐ Fat Free Prepared Popcorn
- ☐ Fig Bars, Whole Wheat, Fat-free, Pride O' the Farm
- ☐ Frozen Fruit Bars
- ☐ Lowfat Cookies, Heaven Scent
- ☐ Meal-in-a-Cup, Dried, Chef's Classics
- ☐ Meal-in-a-Cup, Dried, Fantastic
- ☐ Nonfat Frozen Yogurt (sparingly)
- ☐ Nonfat Granola Bars, Health Valley
- ☐ Imitation Bacon Bits, Soy
- ☐ Spirulina

So What's In a Serving?

According to the Food Guide Pyramid, one serving looks like this:

Bread, Cereal, Rice and Pasta Group:

- 1 slice wholegrain bread
- 1/2 cup cooked rice or pasta
- 1/2 cup cooked cereal
- 1 ounce of ready-to-eat cereal

Fruit Group:

- 1 piece of fruit
- 1 wedge of melon
- 1/4 cup of dried fruit
- 2/3 cup of fruit nectar
- 3/4 cup fresh-squeezed juice (use rarely)

Poultry, Fish, Meat, Eggs, Dried Beans and Nuts Group:

- 2-1/2 to 3 ounces of cooked, skinless turkey or chicken, esp. breast
- 2-1/2 to 3 ounces of cooked lean game meat, or pork tenderloin
- 3 ounces of cooked lean fish
- 1/2 cup of cooked beans
- 2 tablespoons of almond butter (equal to 1/3 serving of meat)
- 1 large egg (equal to 1/2 serving of meat)
- 1/2 cup of nonfat cottage cheese

Vegetable Group:

- 1/2 cup of raw, chopped vegetables
- 1/2 cup of cooked vegetables
- 1 cup of leafy raw vegetables

Note: Eat the maximum number of servings recommended in this group!

Milk, Yogurt and Cheese Group:

- 1 cup of plain yogurt
- 1 cup of acidophilus milk
- 1 cup of regular milk
- 1 cup of soymilk or rice milk
- 1-1/2 to 2 ounces nonfat cheese

Fats, Oils and Sweets:

Limit calories from these, especially if you are trying to lose weight, or balance your blood glucose levels.

Recommendations:

- 1 to 1-1/2 tablespoon, total, daily, use in cooking or as part of a salad dressing *(You will get the most value using oil in an uncooked form!)*

- 1 to 2 tablespoons of sweeteners and fruit preserves, total, daily

- 1 tablespoon of Parmesan or Romano, total, daily

- 1/4 of an avocado 2 or 3 times per week

- 1 cup of organic coffee, maximum per day

So What's On a Label?

The fact is that if you are eating in the fashion outlined in the section entitled "Rules for the Road," you will not need to be so attentive to labels on packages. **Fresh vegetables are fresh vegetables no matter how you slice or dice them!** Except to seek out those which are certified organic, as well as truly *fresh*, there is little else to look for.

The same is true of fresh fruits!

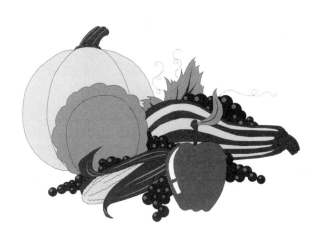

And, except for the wide array of available packaged breads, which may or may not be wholegrain, **a raw, unprocessed,whole grain is exactly that:** *a raw, unprocessed, whole grain*. Just be sure it is *fresh*, and packaged in an *airtight container*. The germ in the whole grain contains oil, which becomes rancid quickly if exposed to oxygen in the air, or if the grain is sitting too long on the shelf. A good rule of thumb is to *buy only amounts that you will use within one to two months*, and *keep them refrigerated* if possible. Definitely keep them in tinted airtight containers away from direct light or sunlight.

Inevitably, if you follow and utilize the **5 Minutes to Health** shopping list, you will be buying some packaged and canned products. However, even those items, included in the list, have been carefully examined and selected, with the objective of providing speed and convenience without sacrificing optimum nutrition and health. And *as long as about 80% of the foods you eat* **are not** *from packages and cans*, and those foods which are from packages and cans are from the shopping list, not only will your total fat intake be low, *it will reflect a very low intake of saturated and hydrogenated fats, as well as cholesterol*, all of which appear to be primary suspects in relationship to raised blood cholesterol levels, heart disease, stroke, cancer, obesity, osteoporosis and arthritis.

Much of the information included on the new food labels, on canned and packaged products, relates to what percentage of the RDI (Reference Daily Intake) you will be getting when you eat a specific amount of that particular item. The RDI's are based on minimum daily requirements for known vitamins and minerals, and maximum recommended allowances for fats (30% of total daily calories), cholesterol (300 mg) and sodium (3300 mg), for **most** normal, healthy people to maintain their health.

But, remember I said earlier in this book, that *when our focus is on eating whole foods in their natural state, we do not need to be counting a lot of numbers and making a lot of calculations.*

And since we are aiming for optimal health, *we are **not** focusing on minimum requirements to maintain health.* Especially if we are not healthy to begin with, and must first build up our health to a level which then readies us for a maintenance program.

Furthermore, I'm suggesting, also, that you strive to keep your *total fat intake* **below** *20% of your total daily calories* (that's about 40 to 50 grams), and your *total sodium intake* **below** *2000 mg per day*. This is easy to do, without any calculations, following the **5 Minutes to Health** plan!

However, there are a few things that are important to be aware of when reading labels. These items are written below as a checklist to assist you at the point of shopping. Good luck!

 ### Check the serving size! If you eat twice as much as the amount listed as a serving size, then you have to realize that you are also getting two times the amount of fat listed, as well as the sodium and cholesterol.

Look at the calories from fat and the total fat grams! A basic rule of thumb is to avoid any foods with more than 2 grams of fat per serving. At 9 calories per gram of fat, this would account for 18 of the total number of calories in a serving. If you have equivalent to 2 servings of an item with 2 grams of fat per serving, then you will get 36 calories from fat.

Now take this a step further! If an item has 500 calories per serving, and lists the calories from fat at 330 calories per serving, you can find the percentage of fat in the product by dividing the 330 calories from fat by the total number of calories in the serving which is 500, and then multiply by 100 to arrive at the percentage of calories from fat in one serving. So, in this case the result is 66%. If we are recommending an upper limit of 20% of our food intake as fat, this food item is way out of line!

The equation for calculation of % fat in an item is:

$$\frac{\text{Total calories of fat}}{\text{Total calories}} \times 100 = \text{\% Calories from Fat}$$

✓   When a label boasts that a product is, for example, 90% Fat Free, 10% Fat, this refers to percent fat by weight, not percent fat by calories. If we have 50 grams of sliced luncheon meat at 90% Fat Free, 5 of those grams are from fat. That's the 10% fat! However, at 9 calories per gram of fat, we have 9 calories X 5 grams, which is 45 calories. If this product has 100 calories, and 45 of them are from fat, we see that 45% of the calories come from fat. So it is obvious that the percent by weight (10% in this example) can be very different from the percent by calories (45%).

✓   **If a food is listed as fat free, sugar or sodium free, or free of calories,** this indicates that only negligible amounts, or absolutely none, of that particular element listed as **"free"** is available in the food.

✓   **Be wary of terms such as "light", "lite" and "low".** These descriptions are somewhat elusive, carrying more than one meaning. It is always best to check the total number of grams or milligrams, in the product, of the specific nutrient in question, e.g., fat, sugar, sodium or cholesterol.

✓   **Be aware, when buying wholegrain bread,** that unless it says specifically "whole wheat," "100% wholegrain," "100% whole wheat," or "Stoneground wholegrain," it is not what you are looking for! *Wheat flour is white flour.* If the bread is brown in color, it is likely molasses or brown sugar that has been added for that purpose. READ THE LABEL!

✓   **The "sugars" number is not necessarily accurate!** Although naturally occurring sugars, eg. fruit sugars and milk sugars are included, the longer-chain sugars, which can account for up to 2/3's of some corn syrups, are omitted.

✓ **Furthermore, there are many names for sugar, besides the word "sugar"!** Basically whenever you see a word on the label which ends with "ose", you can be fairly certain that it is a sugar! To assist you in deciphering sugars in products, I am including a list of terms you may see on a label:

Brown Sugar	Honey
Corn Syrup	Invert Sugar
Corn Syrup Solids	Mannitol
Dextrose (simple sugar)	Molasses
Fructose (fruit sugar)	Natural Sweeteners
Glucose	Raw Sugar
High-Fructose Corn Syrup	Sorbitol
	Sucrose (cane sugar) or Sugar

✓ **And let's go a step further and list the artificial sweeteners which are to avoided!** Remember, only the most natural foods in their most natural states are to be consumed. And artificial sweeteners are anything but natural! So AVOID them.

aspartame includes NutraSweet & Equal

saccharin

acesulfame K includes Sweet One & Sunette

 Choose monounsaturated fats and polyunsaturated fats over saturated fats. And select the least processed, cold-pressed (especially avoid heat processed) varieties, as much as possible.

Avoid anything listed as *"hydrogenated", or "partially hydrogenated"* or products using *vegetable oils which are saturated fats* such as "coconut oil" or "palm oil", "palm kernel oil", or "cocoa butter".

Avoid hard fats such as lard, margarine, and butter. Select butter sprinkles instead! Or try the all natural flavor sprays!

NOTE: As you incorporate more wholesome wholegrain products and fresh organic produce into your diet, you will begin to more fully appreciate their wide variety of unique natural flavors. And, in turn, your need for flavor enhancers eg. butter and fatty spreads will diminish. We only require flavor enhancers to make up for the lack of the original flavor remaining in depleted, over-processed, fabricated foods!

☑ **For the % Daily Value (DV) listed on the food label,** you are being told how much of (in other words, what percentage of) the recommended daily total you will be consuming just from that one food. The basic rule of thumb is: *"If a food has 20% or more of the DV for a particular nutrient, eg. sodium, it is high in that nutrient. If it has 5% or less of a particular nutrient, it is low."* **So to insure a healthy diet, look for foods with a DV of 5 or less for fat, saturated fat, cholesterol and sodium.**

☑ **All ingredients on the label are listed in descending order according to weight.** So, if sugar is the first ingredient in the list, you can bet it makes up the bulk of the product. Therefore, the last item listed makes up the smallest amount of the product by weight.

 As a general guideline for some key dietary components, below you will find listed the daily recommended quantities, as determined by the U.S. Food and Drug Administration:

Total Fat	65 grams or less
Saturated Fat	20 grams or less
Cholesterol	300 milligrams or less
Sodium	2400 milligrams or less
Carbohydrates	at least 300 grams
Fiber	25 grams

This checklist addresses some of the important points to consider for anyone who is very serious about taking charge of his or her own health. *Awareness is the first step* towards making healthy choices. However, **"Awareness without Action" is nothing!** So let's get **active! Read the labels!**

The next step, however, is to go through your cupboards and toss out anything not included in the shopping list. Then stock your shelves and refrigerator with only those foods listed, varying the produce and fish choices each shopping day, and according to season. **Armed with the label information outlined here,** you are now prepared to analyze the items on the shopping list which are packaged or canned.

This may represent a big change in eating habits and lifestyles for many of you. Like any new practice, career, relationship or project, it takes a little getting used to. You may stumble along the way, even fall completely off the wagon. **Whatever you do though, don't beat yourself up!** Remember, you're like a baby learning to walk. It takes time, and a lot of uncertain and unsteady steps, to get it right!

I know, because I've been there and I've done that!! And occasionally, now and then, I give myself permission to eat something higher in fat than I would normally consume. It does the soul and the psyche good to break the pattern a bit. However, I am also reminded at those times, of how much better I feel when my diet is wholesome and natural! Believe me, as time passes, so do the temptations and unhealthy desires. You never want to give up that healthy, alive feeling! Even for a second!

A Well-Equipped Kitchen is
an Efficient Kitchen

Most of us, in an effort to simplify our lives, have kitchens full of equipment and appliances we never use. On one hand, we are very blessed to have so many options available to us. On the other hand, we are cursed! Much of the equipment which was created with the ease of preparation of food in mind, has the added, less attractive feature, of much more work to cleanup after use. So the equipment sits on our shelves, or in our cupboards, until we finally give it away or throw it out!

Taking this into account, the list of items suggested for inclusion in your kitchen, are generally the most user-friendly pieces of equipment and appliances I have been able to assemble over the years. On my own journey to efficiency I've made many mistakes and accumulated many useless pieces of equipment that rarely, if ever, got used.

Therefore, the versatility, as well as ease of cleanup, became important factors in the decision to buy, or not to buy, a particular appliance or piece of equipment.

The following is a basic, but comprehensive, list of those items which have proven, over time, to be the most useful and most versatile items available. When you simplify your food intake, it leads to a simplification of everything else you do in the kitchen as well.

The description of a particular piece of equipment was included only where it was thought to be necessary.

Non-Electrical Equipment:

- 1 set of good quality sharp knives, including utility, paring, slicing and chef's knives
- 2 collapsible steaming baskets, stainless steel
- 2 or 3 cutting boards, preferably dishwasher-safe, plastic, marble, non-porous surface
- 2 sets of measuring spoons
- 2 sets of dry and liquid measuring cups
- 3 to 4 ice-cube trays for freezing pureed fruit, nectars, stocks, water
- Baster
- Broiler pan or broiler pan rack
- Can opener, heavy duty non-electric for easy cleaning after each use
- Canisters, airtight, for grains, pastas, legumes, flour, teabags and loose tea, etc.
- Colander
- Egg-separator, to separate whites from yolks
- Fat separator
- Food scale for weighing foods, eg. fish, poultry and meats
- Food thermometer
- Garlic press
- Hand grater
- Kitchen scissors
- Kitchen timer
- Melon baller
- Nonstick skillets, saucepans, baking pans, cookie sheets -- use nonstick utensils
- Nonstick spatulas and scrapers, regular and slotted
- Paper towels on mounted holder
- Pastry brush
- Plastic wrap and food storage bags
- Popsicle forms for fruit nectar, or pureed fruit, pops
- Pot holders, close to stove, oven, toaster-oven
- Pressure cooker, for long cooking foods, follow manufacturer's directions
- Pyrex oven casserole dishes with lids
- Salad spinner
- Scoops for frozen yogurt, vegetables, coleslaw, etc.
- Sherbet glasses for serving yogurt desserts or fruit salad desserts
- Soup ladel
- Spaghetti lifter
- Tea strainers for loose tea leaves and herbs
- Tongs
- Vegetable brushes for scrubbing vegetables
- Vegetable masher
- Vegetable peeler
- Wire mesh sieve or strainer
- Wire whisks for blending sauces and dips
- Wok, nonstick or stainless steel
- Wooden spoons

Electrical Appliances:

■ Blender -- a more powerful motor is more versatile

■ Blender, handheld -- especially useful when traveling

■ Citrus juicer -- a quick and easy way to juice a lemon or a lime for various uses. A good idea is to use some of the pulp as well, for fiber and bioflavinoids.

■ Coffee-maker -- optional. But if you drink coffee, grind organic coffee beans and prepare the coffee with a good machine to prevent over-cooking it. A coffee-maker can also be used to make herb teas and keep them hot.

■ Coffee mill -- for grinding grains, almonds, organic coffee beans, and whole spices

■ Crockpot or other slow cooker -- takes 3-1/2 to 4-1/2 hours on high setting, and 6 to 9 hours on low setting. Meal can be cooking while you're at work. The taste of some herbs and spices changes in slow cooking, so you may need to adjust types and amounts. Cut vegetables into small, uniform pieces and layer them at bottom of the pot with rest of ingredients on top. Almost impossible to overcook in a crockpot. Do not remove lid during cooking!

■ Hot-air popcorn popper -- fast and easy fluffy, popcorn in minutes. Shake hot popcorn and seasonings together in a brown paper bag or spray the popcorn with all natural flavor sprays.

■ Microwave oven -- optional. An efficient way to reheat foods, it doesn't always produce the best quality product when used for cooking. If you get one, look for a microwave with a 650- to 700-watt output.

■ Mini-chopper / Mini-food processor

■ Rice cooker / Vegetable steamer -- simplifies the cooking of rice, grains and vegetables. Easy to use and easy to clean. Follow the directions that come with it!

■ Toaster oven -- great for open-faced grilled nonfat cheese sandwiches, heating leftovers, toasting large slices of bread, bagels, and rolls, heating tortillas and pita breads, making mini-pizzas, baking potatoes, cooking casseroles, making nonfat nacho plates, etc. Saves on energy bills!

■ Vita-Mix machine, especially the Total Nutrition Center -- the machine of the future, the near future! It mixes, blends, chops, grinds, grates, crushes, purees, liquifies, freezes and cooks food in seconds. In juicing, nothing is thrown away. Cleanup is a snap! The fastest, easiest, and most versatile machine to use, it insures the maintenance of an optimum level of the nutrients originally available in the food. It has almost replaced my blender, coffee grinder, hot plates, chopper and crockpot.

■ Yogurt maker -- best way to get high quality yogurt at a good price. Use certified raw milk or soymilk, and high grade live cultures.

As you can see, **I have not included in my list, a food processor or a juicer, other than the citrus juicer.** For me, the Total Nutrition Center efficiently takes the place of both of these appliances, as well as several others on the list. If you don't have a Vita-Mix machine, but you do have a food processor, by all means use it. The work involved in the cleanup resulted in my own food processor being sold at a yard sale. Also the finished food product just didn't compare with that of the Vita-Mix.

As far as a juicer is concerned, it is an expensive way to throw away all, or most, of the fiber present in our foods, and the nutrients clinging to that fiber! During my own illness, it was not until I began to drink whole food juices, made in the Vita-Mix machine, with nothing thrown out, that my health began to improve. Obviously there was something in the part of the food I was throwing away, when I used the juicer to make juice, that my body required to get well.

The juices, made in the Vita-Mix, are finer in texture and more emulsified, but of course thicker, since every part of the food is included. Simply add more liquid (eg. water, fruit nectar, vegetable broth, low sodium vegetable or tomato juice, etc.) to thin it down to the consistency you prefer. **Once you get used to the taste and consistency of juices made from whole foods, you will never desire the alternatives again!**

Finally, in order to have the most efficient kitchen, it is important to have everything you use within easy reach. **Equipment stored in the cupboard rarely sees the light of day!** So have your equipment and utensils where you can see them and get to them quickly. Keep frequently used utensils in a decorative jar close to the stove and work center of your kitchen. Mount small appliances to the wall or under the cupboards.

30 Menus for Breakfast

MENU 1 ■ Vibrant Fruit Salad ■ Plain Nonfat Yogurt ■ Lemon Zinger Herbal Tea	**MENU 11** ■ High Protein Breakfast Shake	**MENU 21** ■ Berrie Good Kasha ■ Plain Nonfat Yogurt
MENU 2 ■ Raspberry Delight (meal in a glass)	**MENU 12** ■ Fresh Peaches, Sliced ■ Nonfat Cottage Cheese ■ Fat-free Wholegrain Crackers	**MENU 22** ■ Poached Egg/Salsa ■ Nonfat Refried Beans/Grated Nonfat Cheese ■ Corn Tortillas
MENU 3 ■ Nonfat Granola ■ Vanilla Soymilk or Lowfat Acidophilus Milk ■ Fresh Fruit in Season	**MENU 13** ■ Hot 10-Grain Cereal ■ Nonfat Plain Yogurt ■ Ripe Banana/Raisins	**MENU 23** ■ Lowfat Banana Apricot Loaf ■ Nonfat Cottage Cheese and Applesauce Spread
MENU 4 ■ Honeydew Melon ■ Wholegrain Toast ■ Almond Butter	**MENU 14** ■ French Toast/Molly McButter ■ Pure Maple Syrup ■ Bananas and Strawberries	**MENU 24** ■ Toasted Tempeh and Alfalfa Sprout Sandwich ■ Nayonnaise/Sliced Tomato
MENU 5 ■ Brown Rice Pudding ■ Ripe Banana	**MENU 15** ■ Wholegrain Bagel, Toasted ■ Reduced Fat Cream Cheese ■ Fresh Lox ■ Tropical Fruit Salad	**MENU 25** ■ Breakfast Bulgur ■ Lowfat Acidophilus Milk
MENU 6 ■ Spoon-sized Shredded Wheat ■ Vanilla Soymilk or Lowfat Acidophilus Milk ■ Prunes and Apricots, Soaked	**MENU 16** ■ Authentic Muesli ■ Plain Nonfat Yogurt	**MENU 26** ■ Scrambled Tofu and Tomatoes ■ Wholegrain Bagel ■ Butter and Garlic Flavor Spray
MENU 7 ■ Fresh Orange ■ Poached Free-Range Egg ■ Wholegrain Toast ■ Fruit Preserve	**MENU 17** ■ Wheatabix ■ Lowfat Acidophilus Milk ■ Berries and Bananas	**MENU 27** ■ Brown Rice Delight ■ Plain Nonfat Yogurt
MENU 8 ■ Millet Fantasy ■ Plain Nonfat Yogurt	**MENU 18** ■ Oatmeal Pancakes ■ Applesauce/Molly McButter ■ Pure Maple Syrup (optional)	**MENU 28** ■ The Green Machine Shake
MENU 9 ■ Hot Oatmeal, Soaked ■ Soymilk or Nonfat Yogurt ■ Fresh Applesauce	**MENU 19** ■ Fruit Smoothie ■ Potato and Egg Scramble ■ Dark Pumpernickel Bread ■ Fruit Preserves	**MENU 29** ■ Fruity Yogurt ■ Nonfat or Lowfat Wholegrain Muffin
MENU 10 ■ Fresh Fruit Salad ■ Scrambled Egg and Tofu ■ Rye Toast and Fruit Preserves	**MENU 20** ■ Wholegrain English Muffin ■ Ricotta Cheese and Fruit Spread ■ Ginger Tea	**MENU 30** ■ Crazy Mixed-Up Grains ■ Lowfat Acidophilus Milk ■ Apple and Strawberry Sauce

Noteworthy Facts

Do not skip Breakfast! *It is the meal that breaks the fast and raises and maintains your blood sugar level throughout the morning. You need protein, carbohydrates and fats! Fruit, or coffee, alone, won't do it!*

1. Eat only breads listed as *100% Wholewheat, or 100% Wholegrain, or Stoneground*. **Read the Label!** The first ingredient should <u>always</u> be *whole wheat flour*, or another whole grain, not just *wheat flour*.

2. Leftover brown rice, wholegrain or vegetable pasta, or other grains, from the previous lunch or dinner, can be modified for breakfast.

3. Acidophilus milk is a good substitute for yogurt, and generally easier to digest than regular milk, especially for someone experiencing lactose intolerance.

4. One serving of cooked rice or grains, as listed in the breakfast menus on the previous page, is 1 cup, which relates to 2 servings in the Food Guide Pyramid. You can increase or decrease portion size according to your needs.

5. Fresh fruit and plain, nonfat yogurt combinations can be prepared the night before for a breakfast on-the-run, or for a brown bag breakfast or lunch. Carry nonfat granola toppings separately and sprinkle on top just prior to eating, to maintain crispy texture.

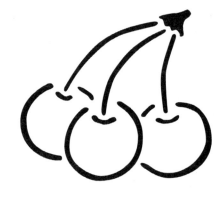

6. Muffins are great for a brown bag breakfast or lunch! But if you buy prepared or packaged muffins, choose those *with no more than 5 grams of fat* and a 100% wholegrain base. *Sugar should not be one of the primary ingredients!* **Avoid** muffin mixes; they are generally higher in sugars and fats than a healthy diet warrants.

7. Use *All Natural Flavor Sprays*, eg. those by Tryson House, or *All Natural Butter Flavored Sprinkles*, eg. Molly McButter and Butter Buds, on toast, or in egg dishes.

30 Menus for Lunch

MENU 1 ■ Split Pea Soup ■ Fresh Organic Salad Mix ■ Nonfat Dressing	**MENU 11** ■ Lentil Vegetable Soup ■ Rye Krisp Crackers ■ Greens and Tomatoes with Dressing	**MENU 21** ■ Fresh Fruit Platter ■ Nonfat Cottage Cheese ■ Nonfat Wholegrain Crackers
MENU 2 ■ Chicken Pita Sandwich ■ Plain Nonfat Yogurt Smoothie	**MENU 12** ■ Turkey Burger with Dijon Mustard ■ Whole Wheat Burger Bun ■ Tomato and Onion Slices	**MENU 22** ■ Lively Chef's Salad ■ High Omega-3 GLA Dressing ■ Whole Wheat Garlic Toast
MENU 3 ■ Tuna Salad Sandwich ■ Fresh Orange	**MENU 13** ■ Mediterranean Potato Salad ■ Frest Fruit Smoothie	**MENU 23** ■ Vegetarian Chili ■ Baked Tortilla Chips ■ Carrots, Celery and Green Peppers
MENU 4 ■ Baked Potato with Skin ■ Nonfat Refried Beans ■ Yogurt and Salsa Topping	**MENU 14** ■ Eggless Egg Salad Sandwich ■ Spinach and Mushroom Salad ■ Peach Nectar	**MENU 24** ■ Bean Burritos with Salsa and Yogurt ■ Mixed Greens and Cherry Tomatoes with Garlic Balsamic Dressing
MENU 5 ■ Turkey Loaf on Whole Wheat Kaiser Roll ■ Tomato and Red Onion Slices	**MENU 15** ■ Nonfat Cheese and Avocado Pita Pocket with Sprouts ■ Fresh Nonfat Banana Yogurt	**MENU 25** ■ Chickpea Spread (Hummus) ■ Whole Wheat Pita ■ Zucchini Salad with Spicy Dressing
MENU 6 ■ Nonfat Cottage Cheese with Peach, Chopped ■ Nonfat or Lowfat Bran Muffin	**MENU 16** ■ Turkey and Tomato on Rye ■ Raw Vegetable Sticks with Yogurt and Salsa Dip	**MENU 26** ■ Curried Lentil Soup ■ Tempeh Sandwich on Sprouted Wholegrain Bread
MENU 7 ■ Minestrone Soup ■ Garlic Pumpernickel Toast ■ Fresh Pear	**MENU 17** ■ Curried Brown Rice Salad ■ Cucumber and Tomato Raita ■ Iced Ginger Tea	**MENU 27** ■ Imitation Crabmeat Salad ■ Baked Potato, Hot ■ Steamed Broccoli and Cauliflower
MENU 8 ■ Wholegrain English Muffin Pizzas ■ Tossed Green Salad ■ Nonfat Mustard Vinaigrette Dressing	**MENU 18** ■ Wholegrain Pasta ■ High Protein Marinara Sauce ■ Mixed Green Salad with Dressing	**MENU 28** ■ Citrus Rice and Bean Salad ■ Lowfat Creamy Cole Slaw
MENU 9 ■ Pasta Salad ■ Wholegrain Bagel ■ Green and Red Seedless Grapes	**MENU 19** ■ Steamed Broccoli, Cauliflower and Carrots with Yogurt Dressing ■ Whole wheat Roll w/Flavored Spray ■ Pineapple and Mango Frappe	**MENU 29** ■ Vegetable-Tofu Medley ■ Brown Rice with Bragg's Liquid Aminos ■ Cucumber and Tomato Raita
MENU 10 ■ Marinated Tofu and Sprout Sandwich ■ Fresh Cantaloupe Half	**MENU 20** ■ Almond Butter, Tomato and Sprouts on Multi-Grain Bread ■ Miso Soup with Tofu Cubes ■ Home-Blended Nonfat Vanilla Yogurt	**MENU 30** ■ Salmon Dill Sandwich on Sprouted Wholegrain Bread ■ Fresh Fruit Salad

Noteworthy Facts

Re-read the notes pertaining to the Breakfast menus!

1. Generally breads are listed in these menus as Wholegrain, versus a specific type, so that you have choice. **Try different varieties to find your own favorites.** As much as possible, **avoid white breads,** including sour dough. Look for breads which begin the listing of ingredients with 100% Wholegrain or Stoneground. Wheat flour is the same as white flour, so don't be fooled by terminology!

2. Lunch is a great time to use up leftover grains, rice or pasta in transportable salads. Simply add:

    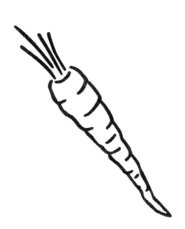

    a. leftover or fresh steamed vegetables

    b. fresh raw vegetables

    c. leftover chicken or turkey breast

    d. leftover fish or shellfish

    e. a nonfat or lowfat seasoned dressing of choice. (See **Dressing** section.)

3. To make garlic toast there are several possible ways, ranging from Lower fat to Low fat to No fat.

    a. Combine 1/2 cup olive oil and 1/2 cup softened butter and whip in blender. Keeps well in refrigerator for about 1 week. Spreads easily. Use sparingly!

    b. Spray toasted bread, bagel, or English muffin with all natural flavor sprays. Tryson House makes several varieties to suit different tastes and needs.

    c. Shake Garlic Molly McButter, or Butter Buds and garlic powder, onto hot toast. For an extra flavor boost, sprinkle grated nonfat cheese onto the garlic toast and grill briefly under the broiler to melt the cheese.

4. **Meat-based lunches are limited in the menus,** providing for an increased intake of high fiber forms of protein, such as the combination of grains and beans (legumes). Contrary to most peoples' understanding, *the meat group includes not only beef, pork, lamb and game meats, but also chicken, turkey, and fish.* The latter varieties are also *flesh foods*, but are generally lower in fat than the former meats listed, especially if the skins are removed.

30 Dinner Menus

MENU 1	MENU 11	MENU 21
■ Baked Chicken Breast ■ Baked Potato w/Yogurt Topping ■ Steamed Broccoli with Butter Sprinkles ■ Frozen Grapes	■ Turkey Loaf w/Mustard Yogurt Dressing ■ Steamed Broccoli with Lemon ■ Garlic Whole Wheat Sourdough Bread ■ Spiced Apple Cider	■ Wholegrain Spaghetti ■ Tofu-Mushroom Marinara Sauce ■ Garlic Whole Wheat English Muffins ■ Frozen Grapes and Banana Chunks
MENU 2 ■ Vegetable and Bean Chili ■ Steamed Brown Rice ■ Mixed Greens and Tomatoes with Buttermilk Dressing ■ Frozen Banana and Date Delight	**MENU 12** ■ Light Whole Wheat Macaroni & Cheese ■ Red and Green Cabbage Slaw ■ Pumpernickel Rolls ■ Fresh Fruit Salad	**MENU 22** ■ Baked Potatoes ■ Tuna and Seasoned Yogurt ■ Steamed Asparagus w/Butter Sprinkles ■ Fresh Cantaloupe
MENU 3 ■ Fettucine Alfredo for Health ■ Caesar Salad with Nonfat Caesar Dressing ■ Fresh Apple and Pear Slices	**MENU 13** ■ Potato and Lentil Soup ■ Romaine, Watercress and Tomato Salad with Dressing ■ Nonfat Wholegrain Crackers ■ Orange Sections	**MENU 23** ■ Salmon Burger on Whole Wheat Kaiser Roll ■ Three Bean Salad ■ Apricot Dream
MENU 4 ■ Baked Potatoes ■ Steamed Broccoli, Cauliflower and Carrots ■ Seasoned Yogurt & Tofu Topping ■ Peaches and Blueberries with Garnish of Nonfat Granola	**MENU 14** ■ Turkey Burger on Wholegrain Roll ■ Tomato and Onion Slices ■ Sweet Potato and Raisin Yogurt Whip	**MENU 24** Evening With Friends: ■ Vegetable Platter ■ Baked Tortilla Chips ■ Variety of Dips ■ Wine Spritzers/Fruit Spritzers
MENU 5 ■ Salad Bar Dinner ■ Nonfat Dressings ■ Heated Wholegrain Rolls with Flavor Spray	**MENU 15** ■ Sweet Potato and Vegetable Casserole ■ Spinach and Tomato Salad with Honey-Lemon Dressing ■ Raspberry-Banana Frappe	**MENU 25** ■ Tofu-Vegetable Frittata ■ Creamy Cabbage Slaw ■ Wholegrain Bagel w/Flavor Spray ■ Pineapple-Almond Whip
MENU 6 ■ Steamed Bulgur w/Nonfat Yogurt ■ Curried Vegetables and Imitation Crabmeat ■ Cucumber and Tomato Raita ■ Blended Frozen Bananas w/Raisins	**MENU 16** ■ Pasta and Vegetable Medley ■ Mixed Green and Red Lettuce with Balsamic Dressing ■ Heated Lowfat Oatmeal Muffin with Blended Fruit Topping	**MENU 26** ■ Steamed Bulgur ■ Curried Chickpeas and Onions ■ Broccoli-Cauliflower Salad ■ Berry-Ricotta Surprise
MENU 7 ■ Turkey Chili ■ Steamed Brown Rice ■ Spinach and Mushroom Salad with Vinaigrette Dressing ■ Whipped Peaches and Almond Yogurt	**MENU 17** ■ Kitchen Sink Salad with Salsa-Yogurt Dressing ■ Whole Wheat Sourdough Bread ■ Brown Rice Pudding with Peaches	**MENU 27** ■ Wholegrain Pasta Primavera ■ Mixed Green Salad w/Herb Dressing ■ Whole Wheat Garlic Toast ■ Fresh Fruit Salad w/Apricot Sauce
MENU 8 ■ Tri-Color Vegetable Pasta and Vegetable Salad (Hot) ■ Tomato and Cucumber Slices with Nonfat Dressing ■ Melon Wedge	**MENU 18** ■ Baked Turkey Breasts ■ Seasoned Baked Potato Wedges ■ Nippy Dijon Coleslaw ■ Whipped Vanilla & Strawberry Yogurt	**MENU 28** ■ Baked Red Snapper with Gingery Pineapple Sauce ■ Seasoned Buckwheat Groats ■ Steamed Kale with Lemon and Butter Sprinkles ■ Cantaloupe Frappe
MENU 9 ■ Fresh Baked Trout ■ Baked Potato with Yogurt Topping ■ Mixed Greens w/Lemon Dressing ■ Whipped Prunes and Almond Yogurt	**MENU 19** ■ Curried Brown Rice, Salmon and Vegetable Salad ■ Marinated Tomato, Onion and Cucumber Slices ■ Mango and Papaya Frappe	**MENU 29** ■ Salmon Loaf with Mustard Sauce ■ Creamy Potato Salad ■ Romaine and Tomato Salad with Lemon-Ginger Dressing ■ Tropical Fruit Yogurt
MENU 10 ■ Fish or Chicken Fajitas ■ Corn Tortillas ■ Mexican Brown Rice ■ Grapes and Melon Slices	**MENU 20** ■ Spicy Beans and Vegetable Stew ■ Steamed Millet ■ Carrot and Celery Sticks ■ Tofu-Yogurt Almond Pudding with Raspberry Puree	**MENU 30** ■ Steamed Brown Rice ■ Spicy Potatoes, Broccoli and Blackeye Peas ■ Raw Veggie Platter with Buttermilk Dip ■ Date and Almond Whip

Noteworthy Facts

1. The Lunch and Dinner menus are interchangeable. **Remember: *Choice* is the key!**

2. The preparation time may take longer in the beginning. But as you become more familiar with this way of eating, and get a handle on the recipes and recipe ideas, you will find your speed picking up. *As you know, you have to crawl before you can walk!*

3. Where a grain is listed as part of the meal, feel free to substitute with any grain you desire, or any prepared grain you have on hand that you want to use up. You can also mix together a variety of grains that you have leftover from previous meals, and create a whole different flavor.

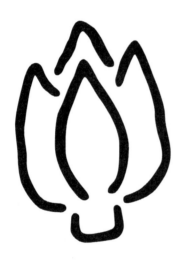

4. Though *I do not recommend cooking with a microwave,* it is a very convenient way to reheat foods, such as grains, potatoes, vegetables or meats, leftover from previous lunches or dinners.

5. In an effort to maintain the aspect of choice as much as possible, salad dressings have not been fully specified for every salad throughout the menus. You can choose from the variety included in the **Salad Dressing** section. You may also choose to substitute one of your favorites for those which have been specified in the menus. Just be sure the dressing you choose is nonfat or very lowfat.

6. An acidophilus-based topping on a main course item, or an acidophilus-based dessert, is incorporated into almost every dinner meal, with the purpose of increasing healthy bacteria in the colon, which in turn, will result in less infections due to a *much stronger and healthier Immune System.*

7. Where breads and rolls are listed, be adventurous! Try different types, varieties and brands. See the notes under Lunch menus for ways to make garlic toast or other flavored breads or toasts.

8.   It is not imperative that you eat the specific vegetables listed in the menus. Simply substitute another vegetable of similar color, texture or variety for the one listed. There is one exception! *Where tomatoes are listed, it is wise to include them, as the Vitamin C in the tomato enhances the iron absorption of the other foods listed in that meal.*

9.   Steamed vegetables may not initially appeal to you in this basic form. However, high fat sauces are not the best solution. Some ideas for dressing up your vegetables include:

- flavor sprays
- butter sprinkles
- lemon juice
- Parmesan or Romano cheese (sparingly)
- Mrs. Dash, Spicy Mrs. Dash, other herb and spice blends
- Bragg's Liquid Aminos
- Tamari sauce
- seasoned yogurt
- salsa
- seasoned vinegars *(avoid white distilled vinegar!)*
- a fresh cilantro and lime combination
- mustard and buttermilk, or yogurt, blends
- horseradish
- hot sauces, eg. Tobasco, Louisiana Hot Sauce and Jalapeno pepper sauces.

10.   If you have a tendency to eat too much at meals, it may be helpful for you to begin your lunch and dinner meals with a broth-based soup, that can be made simply by adding about 1 tsp. - 1 tbsp. of a base to a cup of hot or boiling water. Some base ideas include:

- Bragg's Liquid Aminos
- Gayelord Hauser's All Natural Instant Vegetable Broth
- Bernard Jensen's Vegetable Broth and Seasoning Powder
- Red Miso Paste
- Hatcho Miso Paste
- Marmite vegetable paste
- Take 5 Vegetable Powder (has lemony flavor)

All of those listed are natural, wholesome products without added salt, sugar or MSG. They can be used as a *hot beverage* to replace coffee, or as a *soup base*, or as a *seasoning* in cooked or raw foods.

Other seasonings, chopped vegetables, tofu cubes, or leftover grains or beans, can be added to these soup blends to give a real zingy flavor, or more sustenance.

11.   It is wise to make up a large amount of some of your favorites, eg. the soups, stews, chilis, or meatloaves, as these are very versatile items that lend themselves to a multitude of different meal combinations. For example, the turkey chili:

- chili and brown rice
- sloppy joe on wholegrain roll
- chili over vegetable pasta
- chili and grains mixed, as a casserole, with lowfat cheese topping
- chili burritos on corn or whole wheat tortillas
- baked potato topped with chili and nonfat or lowfat cheese
- thinned with vegetable stock, and rice and vegetables added, for soup

This is your opportunity to be creative. Give it your best shot!

12.   Beverages, other than fruit frappes, have not been listed with the meals. If you look under the section **"Let's Drink to Our Health,"** which lists the wonderful variety of drink and beverage possibilities, you can try them all to determine which ones you enjoy the most and will continue to use. Remember, variety is the spice of life, so don't get stuck in a rut, using only one or two of the choices. *There is no excuse for boredom with such a selection!*

Quick and Easy Recipes and Food Preparation Hints

The goal of the following recipes is to provide the highest level of nutrition, with the most enjoyable flavor, in the least amount of time. Generally, only items which require a minimum number of steps in their preparation are included. Overall, my philosophy is, *if it can't be done in 5 minutes, it won't be done by me!*

Throughout this section the objective has been to provide all of the information necessary to make incorporation of the 30-day menus, for breakfasts, lunches and dinners, a snap. Apart from the actual recipes for the specific menu items, wherever appropriate, further suggestions and ideas are included to assist you in widening the variety of options you have. Some recipes actually lend themselves to the substitution of particular ingredients, with other ingredients, which in turn can result in a different flavor or texture, or both.

Also, if you do not like a particular ingredient in a specific recipe, either omit it or substitute it with something else. For example, if a shake recipe calls for a banana, and a banana is the one fruit you detest, change it to a fruit you love, such as a peach or a pear. Remember what I said about being adventurous! And now, with all of the right foods stocked in your cupboards and refrigerator, preparing healthy meals **will** be a snap. So go for it and have lots of fun doing it!

In order to ease your shift towards a less meat-oriented diet,
the directions for buying, storing and preparing the various grains and legumes, have been presented in user-friendly chart forms, that you can copy and attach to your refrigerator with a magnet, for easy reference. For your interest, some pertinent nutrition information is also included.

With respect to the amounts and types of seasonings used in the recipes,
please understand that these are only suggestions. Nothing is carved in stone! Because everyone's taste buds are different, you may want to experiment to find your own most desired flavors. **This is your opportunity to be the creator!** Start with what is recommended in the specific recipe, and adjust it until you get it the way you want it. And remember that fresher herbs and spices are more potent in flavor than those which have been sitting on your shelf for awhile, so use less.

You will notice throughout the Recipes Section, *there are spaces included for notes* for your convenience. Here, you can list all of the changes you may have made to a recipe, so that it is more in line with your tastes. Whenever you use that recipe in the future, your changes will be right at your fingertips. You won't have to go through the trial and error stage again and again. And you won't have to waste time searching for those notes you made on that loose piece of scrap paper that somehow got lost in the shuffle!

And a final note:

If you want to find a particular recipe in a hurry, look it up in the **Recipe Index** at the end of the book. In the **Contents** page, at the front of the book, it will be listed under the heading that best describes the menu item, e.g., Salad Dressings, Marinades, Breakfast Entrees, etc.

So let's get started!

On your mark, get set...

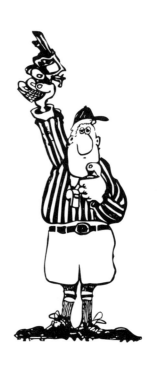

The Scoop on Beans and Lentils!

Shopping Tips:
- Buy large packages of dried beans.
- Buy canned beans for convenience.
- Try different types of beans -- be adventurous!
- Generally 1 lb. of dry beans equals 2 cups, or 6 cups cooked.
- One 16 ounce can of beans equals 2 cups cooked.

Storage Tips:
- Avoid storing at high temperatures and humidity.
- Store in cool, dry, dark place.
- Keep in air-tight and moisture-proof jars or containers.
- Drain cooked beans while hot; store in refrigerator or freezer.
- Drain and rinse canned beans before storing.
- Drained liquid can be stored separately; add to beans later.
- Dry beans properly stored keep indefinitely.
- Cooked beans keep up to 1 week in refrigerator.
- Cooked beans keep up to 1 year in freezer.

Nutrition Points:
- Combined with wholegrains, beans are a good protein source.
- Complex carbohydrates contribute to sustained energy levels.
- High dietary fiber maintains a healthy colon and digestive tract.
- B vitamins protect the nervous system and turn food into energy.
- Iron builds healthy red blood cells.
- Potassium is important for regulation of body fluid balance.
- Calcium and phosphorus form basis of strong bones and teeth.
- Copper, magnesium, manganese, zinc are for metabolic processes.
- Beans are low in fat, cholesterol and sodium (unless canned).

Cleaning Beans:
- Wash dry beans thoroughly, removing bad beans and objects.
- Drain and rinse canned beans thoroughly to reduce sodium.

Soaking Dry Beans:
- Overnight: Add 6 to 8 cups cold water to 1 lb. of beans. Let stand overnight at a cool room temperature. Drain and rinse, discarding the soak water.
- Quick soak: Add 6 to 8 cups hot water to 1 lb. of beans. Bring water to a boil and cook for 2 to 3 minutes. Set pot of beans aside, covered, for 1 to 2 hours.

Cooking Beans:
- Drain and rinse soaked beans after either soaking method.
- Place beans in a large pot and cover with 6 cups hot water.
- Simmer beans until they are tender, keeping the pot lid tilted.
- Essential to flavor are long, slow cooking and low temperatures.
- Add water as necessary to keep beans covered while cooking.

Bean Facts:
- Cooking too fast at high temperatures splits the skins.
- Hard water or high altitude increase soaking and cooking times.
- A tablespoon of olive oil added during cooking reduces foaming.
- Acidic ingredients slow down cooking, so add tomatoes, lemon or lime juice, vinegar, wine, etc. at end of cooking.
- Baking soda results in a loss of vitamins, so avoid using it.
- Salt toughens bean skins and slows cooking, so add when beans are almost tender.
- Lentils, red, brown or green, do not require presoaking.
- For convenience, soak and cook a double batch of beans, and freeze 1/2 of it for future use.
- The flavor of any seasonings added during cooking, develops more fully if beans are prepared the day before.
- Beans and lentils can be added to salads, soups, stews, stir-fries, and casseroles, or made into dips and sandwich spreads.
- Drained liquid from cooked beans can be used as a base for soups or stews, to steam vegetables, or added to casseroles.
- Mashed beans can be used to thicken soups and stews.

Cooking Times:

Azuki (adzuki) beans	1½ - 2 hours
Black beans	2 - 2½ hours
Black-eyed peas	30 - 45 minutes
Chick-peas	3 - 4 hours
Great Northern beans	2½ - 3 hours
Green peas, whole	60 - 75 minutes
Kidney beans	2 - 2½ hours
Lentils	40 - 60 minutes
Lima beans	40 - 75 minutes
Marrow beans	2½ - 3 hours
Navy beans	2 - 2½ hours
Pea beans	3 - 3½ hours
Pinto beans	2 - 2½ hours
Red beans, small	3 - 3½ hours
Roman beans	2 - 2½ hours
Soybeans	3 - 3½ hours
Split peas	45 - 60 minutes
White beans, small	3 - 3½ hours

** These are approximate times only. Generally beans are done when the skins begin to break and the beans are tender throughout. Check for tenderness by biting into a bean.

The Scoop on Grains!

Shopping Tips:
- Buy only fresh grains, as high fat content in germ of wholegrains turns rancid quickly.
- Buy from stores and mail-order houses with a high turnover.
- Small amounts bought as needed, is the rule of thumb.
- Purchase vacuum-packed or sealed packages instead of scooping and bagging your own from a large open container.

Storage Tips:
- Keep in air-tight and moisture-proof jars or containers.
- Store in a cool, dark place preferably the refrigerator.
- Stored properly and in the refrigerator most will keep up to 6 mo.
- Stored properly but in a cupboard, most will keep up to 2 months, unless in a hot climate, or a hot season.
- Store cooked leftover grains in air-tight container up to 3 days in refrigerator, or up to 6 months in freezer.

Nutrition Points:
- Combined with legumes, grains are a good protein source.
- Complex carbohydrates contribute to sustained energy levels.
- High dietary fiber maintains a healthy colon and digestive tract, and contributes to lowering of blood cholesterol.
- B vitamins protect the nervous system and turn food into energy.
- Magnesium assists muscle and nerve functions, and regulates blood pressure.
- Iron builds healthy, oxygen-rich red blood cells.
- Zinc is essential for wound-healing and proper immune function.
- Vitamin E is a natural immune-system booster.
- Grains are low in fat, cholesterol and sodium.

Cleaning Grains:
- Always rinse wholegrains in cool, running water before cooking.
- Bulgur and couscous are exceptions; they turn soggy if rinsed.

Cooking Grains:
- Couscous and bulgur are fluffier when soaked in boiling water for about 15 to 20 minutes, instead of cooking.
- For other grains, bring water to a boil and add the grain.
- Bring to simmer, cover and cook for appropriate amount of time.
- Avoid stirring while cooking; it makes most grains sticky.
- Cornmeal (or polenta) is cooked uncovered and stirred often.
- General Rule, 2 cups water to 1 cup dry grain, except cornmeal at 4 cups water, and brown rice and barley at 3 cups water.

Grain Facts:

- Flavor of most grains, especially millet, is enhanced by roasting lightly in a dry skillet prior to cooking.
- Use vegetable broth or juice, or fruit nectar or juice, instead of water for cooking.
- Add chopped onions and garlic during cooking process.
- Leftover grains can be used as the base for a salad, added to soups, stews, and casseroles, made into healthy puddings, added to protein shakes, or eaten as is with a dressing.
- Grains can be ground to a finer texture or a powder, in a coffee mill or blender, and used to coat fish or chicken.
- Ground dry grains can be used to thicken soups, stews, sauces, and dips, or added to health drinks.
- Prepare "cooked" ground grains, individually or mixed, by soaking ground grains briefly (about 20 minutes) in hot water, or lemon juice, or a combination of both; then serve.

Cooking Times:

Barley	1 - 1½ hours
Brown Rice	30 - 45 minutes
Buckwheat (kasha)	15 - 20 minutes
Bulgur (cracked wheat)	15 - 20 minutes
Cornmeal (polenta)	15 - 20 minutes
Couscous	10 - 12 minutes
Millet	20 - 30 minutes
Oatmeal	7 - 15 minutes
Quinoa	12 - 15 minutes
Wheat Berries	1½ - 2 hours

**These are approximate times only. Follow directions on the package. Cook or soak the grain until desired consistency. It is best to let the grain sit covered for a few minutes after cooking. Then fluff with a fork.

Cooking with Herbs and Spices (Seasoning Without Salt)

Apart from the individual herbs and spices listed here, there are many herb and spice *blends* available, which are also handy to have in your spice cupboard. The label on the bottle or container outlines the many uses for the particular blend. Be adventurous and try some of them.

However, some points to remember when purchasing individual herbs and spices, or the blends:

a.   Buy only small amounts of each item to insure freshness and full flavor enhancement. Keep only 6 months, at most 1 year, and then discard.

b.   Buy organic whenever possible. At the very least, shop for herbs and spices in ethnic grocery stores, where they are often at their freshest!

c.   Avoid irradiated herbs and spices! The label on packaged seasonings will tell you if they are. Look in Wholefood and Health Food Stores.

d.   With the blends, avoid anything with MSG or excessive amounts of salt, if any.

e.   To interchange fresh herbs for dried, use 3 to 5 times more fresh than dried.

f.   Allow the flavor of herbs and spices in salad dressings to develop, by letting the mixture sit for at least 15 minutes prior to serving.

g.   For long-cooking soups, stews and sauces, add the seasonings during the last 30 minutes of cooking. Prolonged cooking dissipates flavor.

h.   To reduce salt intake, substitute strong, flavorful seasonings such as garlic, onion, black pepper, cayenne pepper, chili powder, curry, cumin, basil, or oregano.

i   To release the flavor of dried herbs, crumble them before adding to the dish.

j.   Toasting whole spices briefly in a heavy, dry skillet just before using them, intensifies their flavor.

k.   Many herbs and spices are very powerful, so go slow. Experiment until you find the amount that's right for your taste buds!

l.   If you add too much to a particular dish, doctor the dish with unseasoned grains, rice, extra potatoes, or more of all of the ingredients. Or serve the dish chilled!

Cooking with Herbs and Spices (continued)

Name	Culinary Uses
Allspice	casseroles, curries, rich soups, carrots, tomatoes, squash, eggplant, sweet potatoes, marinades, desserts, fruit pie, pumpkin pie
Anise	soups, stews, casseroles, fruit salads, vegetable salads, poultry, breads, cakes, cookies, applesauce, apple pie
Bay Leaf	marinades, soups, stews, stuffings, sauces, fish, poultry, tomato juice, tomato soup, sauces for cooked greens, dressings for raw greens, meat, roasts
Basil	tomatoes, tomato sauces, eggs, cheese dishes, dips, curries, soups, salad dressings, sauces, marinades, vegetables, fish, poultry, game meats, appetizers, pizza, Italian cooking, Mediterranean cooking
Capers	sauces, gravies, salads, salad dressings, canapes, tomato dishes, eggplant dishes, fish dishes
Caraway	cabbage, carrots, green beans, potatoes, sauerkraut, cabbage soups, borscht, goulash-type stews, breads
Cardamon	marinades, curries, cabbage, fish, poultry, pork tenderloin, coffee, spiced punches, pies, cakes
Cayenne	egg dishes, cheese dishes, fish, salads, soups, sauces, stews, curries, dressings, Mexican cooking. **NOTE:** Helps to prevent flatulence from gaseous vegetables.
Celery Seed	soups, stews, salads, stuffings, vegetable dishes, potato salad, cole slaw, egg salad, tuna salad, fish dishes, game meat dishes, breads
Chervil	cream soups, stews, sauces, salad dressings, egg salads, chicken dishes, fish dishes. **NOTE:** Loses flavor when used in cooking.
Chicory	salads, coffee substitute
Chives	cold soups, salads, dips, eggs, yogurt, potatoes, cabbage, vegetable dishes, fish dishes, chicken dishes. **NOTE:** Loses flavor when used in cooking.
Cinnamon	eggplant, squash, tomatoes, carrots, apples, chicken and game meats cooked with fruit, pork tenderloin, cakes, pies, spiced beverages
Cloves	marinades, pickled fruits, pickled vegetables, cakes, cookies, spiced beverages
Coriander	marinades, curries, fish, game meat dishes, relishes, yogurt desserts, pickles, spicy punches, coffee, cakes, breads

62

Cumin   rice dishes, curries, dips, spaghetti sauce, chilis, salads, sauerkraut, yogurt dishes, tofu dishes, spicy vegetables, spicy game meats, Indian cooking, Mexican cooking

Curry (a blend)   rice dishes, curries, dips, yogurt dishes, spicy vegetables, spicy fish, chicken or game meats, lentil dishes, Indian cooking, Oriental cooking, ginger dishes

Dandelion   lentils, omelettes, soups, salads, sandwiches, vegetables, breads, coffee substitute, jellies

Dill   soups, sauces, salads, vegetables, potatoes, carrot salads, cucumbers (especially pickled), green beans, cabbage, sauerkraut, fish (especially salmon), shellfish, yogurt, eggs, cottage cheese, rice dishes

Fennel   soups, stews, sauces, salads, vegetables, sweet potatoes, spicy game meats, fish, oily fish, seafood sauces, pizza, breads, cakes

Fenugreek   curries, stews, spice mixtures, chutneys, yogurt puddings, baked goods, breads, sweet sauces

Garlic   marinades, dips, salad dressings, soups, sauces, salads, egg dishes, cheese dishes, vegetable dishes, fish, poultry, Italian cooking. **NOTE:** 1/4 tsp. of garlic powder = 1 small clove of garlic

Garam Masala (a blend)   soups, stews, dressings, vegetable stews and dishes, seafood dishes, tofu dishes, yogurt dips, yogurt drinks

Ginger   marinades, curries, ginger tea, salads, horseradish dips, cocktail sauces, mustards, relishes, salad dressings, appetizers, oily fish, clams, seafood, Oriental cooking

Horseradish   dips, cocktail sauces, mustards, relishes, salad dressings, appetizers, oily fish, clams, seafood

Lovage   soups, stews, sauces, casseroles, chowders, omelettes, salads

Marjoram   soups, stews, stuffings, sauces, salads, eggplant, tomatoes, Brussels sprouts, carrots, spinach, zucchini, mushrooms, squash, fish, fowl, pork tenderloin, egg dishes, cheese dishes, Mediterranean cooking

Mint/Spearmint   cold soups (especially fruit), fruits, beans, carrots, eggplant, peas, potatoes, spinach, yogurt dishes, strong-flavored fish, cheese dishes, cheese balls, teas, beverages, desserts

Mustard   soups, stews, sauces, dips, salad dressings, cheese dishes, eggs, potato dishes, onion dishes, tofu dishes

Nutmeg   eggplant, squash, tomatoes, carrots, applesauce, chicken and game meats cooked with fruit, cheese dishes, spicy punches, cookies, pies, breads

Onion   marinades, soups, stews, sauces, dips, salads, stuffing, vegetable dishes, egg dishes, cheese dishes, fish, poultry, game meats

Oregano   soups, stews, salads, stuffings, tomatoes, tomato sauces, peppers, summer squash, zucchini, beans, eggs, pasta dishes, pizza sauces, pork tenderloin, game meats, Italian, Greek and Mexican cooking

Paprika   soups, stews, chilis, Hungarian goulash, sauces, eggs dishes, cheese dishes, potatoes, pasta dishes

Parsley   soups, stews, sauces, salads, stuffings, vegetable and salad garnish, tomato dishes, potato dishes, cheese dishes

Pepper   all purpose spice, preservative (especially for meats)

Poppy Seed   marinades, dressings, stuffings, fruit dishes, yogurt desserts, cottage cheese blends, breads, cakes

Rosemary   marinades, sauces, stews, gravies, pea soup, beans, carrots, squash, peas, cauliflower, rice dishes, poultry, fish, pork tenderloin, fish and poultry stuffing, vegetable dishes, breads

Saffron   rice dishes, poultry dishes, fish dishes, breads, cakes, Spanish cooking eg. Paella

Sage   soups, chowders, stews, sauces, stuffings, eggplant, onions, tomatoes, lima beans, omelettes, herb cheese, fish, game meats, pork tenderloin, duck, coffee and tea substitute

Savory   soups, stews, salads, stuffings, beans, green peas, pea soup, oily fish, game meat dishes, pork tenderloin

Tarragon   egg dishes, omelettes, Bearnaise sauce, tartar sauce, fish, poultry, salad dressings, vinegar, French cooking

Thyme   creamy soups, clam chowder, stews, sauces, stuffings, beans, beets, carrots, mushrooms, onions, potatoes, tomatoes, summer squash, green vegetables, fish, poultry, game meats, pork tenderloin

Turmeric   curries, rice dishes, salad dressings, dips, egg dishes, tofu dishes, Indian cooking

Vanilla/Mexican   shakes, yogurt desserts, sweet yogurt dips, rice dishes, rice

Vanilla   Vanilla pudding, breakfast grains, sweet sauces, milk drinks and milk desserts

Versatile Tofu: The Culinary Chameleon

Tofu is one of those rare foods that can be added to virtually any dish to enhance the protein content, without adding a distinctive flavor of its own. It simply takes on the flavors and seasonings of anything it is cooked or prepared with.

Tofu, also called *bean curd*, is a protein-rich food, which is low in calories, sodium, and fat, especially saturated fat, has no cholesterol, and is relatively inexpensive. It comes in several versatile forms, from **soft or silken**, to **firm**, to **extra-firm**, making it an excellent product for thickening, extending, adding to soups, stews, salads, egg or vegetable dishes, or as a main dish item.

In recipes calling for cream, cream cheese, cottage cheese, ricotta cheese, or eggs, tofu can be substituted. *A one-to-one ratio is a good substitution standard.*

This wonderfully versatile food can be cubed, diced, crumbled or pureed. It can be an obvious ingredient in a recipe, or camouflaged by the other ingredients or flavors.

You will find several recipe ideas in this book. But apart from actual recipes, there are many quick-fix possibilities which incorporate tofu for the purpose of increasing the protein content, and therefore, the sustained satiety value (satisfied feeling after eating) of a meal; a meal which may otherwise have left you feeling hungry an hour after eating it.

So here's a list of suggestions! Try them. And then create your own!

1.   Blend 1/2 cup of soft tofu into a healthy breakfast shake, or a milk shake.

2.   Blend soft tofu, plain yogurt, fruit and maybe a teaspoon of pure maple syrup together into a dessert pudding.

3.   Blend or mash, soft or firm tofu into savory or sweet dips.

4.   Marinate 1/4 inch thick slices of firm or extra-firm tofu, in a blend of tamari sauce, garlic, ginger, minced capers, green onions and organic cider vinegar, overnight, and then:

     a.   use as a sandwich base, with lettuce, alfalfa sprouts and tomatoes
     b.   cut into cubes to toss into a chef's salad
     c.   add to scrambled eggs, egg salad, or omelettes
     d.   add to potato salad, or potato-based casseroles
     e.   cut into cubes and toss over brown rice, or other grains
     f.   serve as a main dish entree with steamed vegetables

      g.   place a slice in a baked potato, and top with a yogurt and chive dressing
      h.   use as a base for a pita pocket sandwich with a thin hummus dressing
      i.   toss cubes into a basic miso broth
      j.   crumble or finely dice, the tofu slices over steamed vegetables

5.   Add cubes of tofu to vegetable or bean, soups or stews, to increase protein content after soups or stews are finished cooking. DO NOT COOK TOFU!

6.   Add cubes of firm tofu, or mashed soft tofu, to any casserole dish.

7.   Mash soft tofu into basic non-meat marinara sauce for added sustenance. Add after cooking is completed.

8.   Chop firm tofu into marinara sauce for a chunkier texture. Add after cooking is completed.

9.   To top a baked potato, puree 1/2 cup of soft tofu, and blend with juice of 1 lemon and 1 tbsp. chives.

10.   Serve slices of extra-firm tofu with low sodium soy sauce, or Bragg's Liquid Aminos, for breakfast, or lunch on wholegrain toast.

11.   For a creamy vegetable soup, blend tofu with reheated leftover vegetable soup.

12.   For a cold, creamy fruit soup, blend tofu, vanilla soymilk, frozen berries and a banana together, and sprinkle cinnamon on top of each serving.

Another food, which deserves honorable mention here, is tempeh.

It is also a very versatile high-protein cultured food, made from soybeans and sometimes grains. Though most tempehs are flavorful to begin with, they adapt very well to many of the suggestions outlined above for tofu, especially the more savory combinations.

This unique food is also adaptable to the use of marinades. Tempeh, like tofu, can be marinated in the combination of ingredients outlined in Suggestion #4, and served in the various ways listed for marinated tofu.

Tempeh is available in a variety of flavors. So don't be shy! Try them all to find the flavors you most enjoy. Experiment with different ways of serving this nutritious alternative to meat. *Your body will thank you for giving it such high-powered nutrition without all of the additional saturated fats and chemicals present in most of our meat-based products.*

30 Quick Toppings for
Baked Potatoes, Brown Rice, Wholegrains

1. Nonfat, plain yogurt with chives.

2. Nonfat yogurt and salsa -- equal parts.

3. Nonfat vegetarian chili topped with nonfat grated cheddar cheese.

4. Steamed broccoli and cauliflower over potato, topped with nonfat yogurt.

5. Blended, heated, marinara sauce and soft tofu, sprinkled with Parmesan cheese.

6. Nonfat vegetarian refried beans, or any seasoned beans, blended until smooth.

7. Blend of chopped onions, mushrooms, and tuna.

8. Lentil and vegetable soup, topped with a dollop of nonfat yogurt.

9. Salsa topped with grated nonfat cheese, and melted under the broiler.

10. Blended yogurt and lowfat ricotta cheese with dill and chives.

11. Equal blend, with either a blender or a fork, of yogurt, cottage cheese and salsa.

12. Cottage cheese blended until smooth with minced red peppers, ginger and olives.

13. Yogurt blended with ginger, cumin and celery seed.

14. Nonfat yogurt blended with minced parsley and a small portion of blue cheese.

15. Lowfat ricotta cheese mixed with capers and imitation bacon bits.

16. Scrambled egg and tofu mixture topped with salsa.

17. Nonfat yogurt seasoned with minced garlic, onions, celery and Spicy Mrs. Dash.

18. Garlic Molly McButter and nonfat yogurt.

19. Nonfat yogurt and almond butter blended with jalapeno peppers.

20. Nonfat yogurt mixed with chopped prunes and almonds.

21. Nonfat yogurt and red caviar.

22. Lowfat ricotta cheese and sardines blended.

23. Blended soft tofu, raisins, almonds and Tabasco sauce.

24. Blended broccoli, cauliflower, onions, garlic and nonfat yogurt, or buttermilk.

25. Blended buttermilk, ricotta cheese, Spicy Mrs. Dash and imitation bacon bits.

26. Leftover chili, vegetable stew, chicken stew, soups and steamed vegetables.

27. Mashed avocado, chopped tomatoes, onions and garlic mixed with yogurt.

28. Mashed avocado and salsa mixed with nonfat cottage cheese or lowfat ricotta.

29. Blended tempeh, nonfat yogurt, and salsa.

30. Chopped tempeh, onions, minced garlic, fresh lemon juice and Tabasco sauce.

NOTE: Though it is not always written, it must be understood that any yogurt, ricotta cheese or cottage cheese used, is of the nonfat or lowfat variety. These toppings are designed to be high enough in protein to make the baked potato, or grain, a meal. Just add a salad, with a nonfat dressing, to complete the meal.

Breakfast Recipes

Vibrant Fruit Salad

1 medium peach, chopped
1 medium orange, in sections
1/4 of a fresh pineapple, chopped
6 strawberries, sliced
1 medium banana, sliced

1/2 cup plain, nonfat yogurt
1/4 tsp. raspberry extract
2 tsp. pure maple syrup
2 tbsp. unsweetened shredded coconut

1.   Blend the yogurt, maple syrup and extract together.
2.   Fold in all of the prepared fruit, including any juice from the pineapple.
3.   Serve in your most elegant glass dessert dishes.
4.   You may top with additional plain, nonfat yogurt.
5.   Sprinkle shredded coconut on the top of each serving.

Variation: Can substitute any in-season fruit.

Makes 2 servings

Raspberry Delight: Healthy Shake

2 cups vanilla soymilk, chilled
1 cup fresh raspberries, chilled
1 medium banana
1 - 2 tbsp. untoasted wheatgerm

1/4 tsp. almond extract
2 tsp. spirulina powder
1 - 2 tsp. pure maple syrup (optional)

1.   Blend all ingredients together in a blender or a Vita-Mix machine.
2.   If not sweet enough, add 1 - 2 tsp. pure maple syrup.

Note: If made in a Vita-Mix machine, the texture and blend are much smoother and finer. However blend for only a few seconds to avoid heating the product, as the power of the motor generates heat while it blends. To counteract this heating action, simply add 3 or 4 ice cubes with the other ingredients, during the blending process.

Makes 2 servings.

Brown Rice Pudding

A great way to use up leftover cooked brown rice!

1 cup cooked brown rice, chilled	1/4 tsp. fresh ginger, grated
1/2 cup plain, nonfat yogurt	2 tbsp. unsulphured raisins
1/2 cup vanilla soymilk	2 tsp. pure maple syrup
1/2 tsp. cinnamon	4 almonds, chopped

1. Mix all of the ingredients together.
2. Can be served heated (not to boiling point) or chilled.

Note: If served chilled, it is best prepared the night before and stored, covered, in the refrigerator. This allows for the flavors to marinate more fully. To maintain the texture of the almonds, add them just prior to serving.

Makes 1 - 2 servings

Notes:

Hot Oatmeal, Soaked

1/2 cup old fashioned oats
1/2 inch fresh ginger, ground
Boiling water
1 - 2 tbsp. wheatgerm or bran
1 cup vanilla soymilk or plain, nonfat yogurt

1 tsp. cinnamon
2 tbsp. unsulphured raisins
1 medium unpeeled apple, chopped
2 tsp. sucanat (optional)

1. Grind oatmeal and ginger together into a powder, in a coffee mill or Vita- Mix machine.
2. Cover the oatmeal and ginger with boiling water. Let sit for 20 minutes.
3. Mix in the wheatgerm, cinnamon, raisins, apple and sucanat.
4. Top with either soymilk, or yogurt, or a combination of the two.

Note: Actually this oatmeal will only be warm by the time you eat it, as prepared above. If you desire hot oatmeal, simply reheat it in a microwave oven, just prior to serving. Or sit the covered bowl of oatmeal and ginger over a pot of very hot water during the 20 minute soaking period.

Variations: 1. Substitute any other dried fruit for the raisins.
2. Substitute any fresh ripe fruit for the apple.
3. The oatmeal and ginger can be soaked together in an unground form, and then blended in a blender or Vita-Mix machine, after the soaking period, just prior to the addition of the remaining ingredients.

Makes 2 servings

Millet Fantasy

1/2 cup millet, uncooked
Boiling water
1/2 cup vanilla soymilk
1/2 tsp. cinnamon
1 medium peach or banana, chopped

1 tbsp. unsulphured dates, chopped
3 almonds, chopped
1 - 2 tsp. pure maple syrup
1/2 cup nonfat plain yogurt

1. Grind the millet to a powder in either a coffee mill or a Vita-Mix machine.
2. Cover the millet with boiling water. Let sit for 20 minutes. *A great opportunity to get ready for the day ahead!*
3. Mix the maple syrup and yogurt together. Let sit while you prepare the rest.
4. Mix the soymilk and cinnamon into the soaked millet.
5. Add the chopped fruit, dates and almonds.
6. Top with nonfat yogurt.

Makes 1 - 2 servings

Fresh Fruit Salads

Below are some suggestions for combinations of fruit for fruit salads. It is always best to use fruits which are in season. Each combination is approximately 2 servings.

ONE
1 medium banana, sliced
1 cup green seedless grapes
1 medium green apple, chopped

TWO
1 cup fresh pineapple, chopped
1 mango, cubed
1 medium banana, sliced

THREE
1 cup cantaloupe, cubed
1 cup honeydew melon, balled
1/2 cup watermelon, chopped

FOUR
1 medium banana, sliced
1 medium peach, chopped
1 medium pear, in thin wedges

FIVE
1 papaya, chopped
1/2 cup fresh pineapple, chopped
1/2 medium avocado, diced

SIX
1 medium banana, sliced
1 medium nectarine, in thin wedges
1 medium peach, chopped

SEVEN
1 papaya, diced
1 mango, diced
1 cup fresh cherries
1 medium banana, sliced

EIGHT
1 medium pear, diced
1 medium orange, in wedges
1 medium grapefruit, in wedges
1/2 cup fresh pineapple, cubed

NINE
2 medium bananas, sliced
1/2 medium avocado, sliced
1/4 - 1/2 tsp. cinnamon

TEN
1 cup fresh strawberries, sliced
1/2 cup fresh raspberries
1/2 cup fresh blueberries

Any of the above combinations can be served plain, or with nonfat yogurt dressings, or sprinkled with fresh squeezed lemon juice, or with shredded almonds or coconut, or topped with a few sunflower, or pumpkin, or sesame seeds, or any combinations of these ingredients.

Notes: _____

Fresh Applesauce

1 apple, unpeeled, cored   1 - 2 tsp. pure maple syrup
1/2 tsp. cinnamon   1 - 2 tbsp. pure apple cider (optional)

1.   Process in blender for about 30 seconds or Vita-Mix machine for about 10 seconds.
2.   Can add a little pure apple cider, to thin it down or for added flavor.

Makes 1 - 2 servings

Prunes and Apricots for Topping on Cereal

1/2 cup of dried prunes, unsulphured
1/2 cup of dried apricots, unsulphured
Boiling water

1.   Just cover with boiling water, in the same bowl, the dried prunes and dried apricots.
2.   Cover the bowl with a thick tea towel. Let sit overnight.
3.   Serve 3 - 4 pieces of fruit, and some of the soaking liquid, per person, on the cereal.
4.   Refrigerate the undrained fruit, in a covered container, for future use. Use all of the product within 1 week.

Notes: _____

Scrambled Egg and Tofu

Olive oil or canola oil-based spray
4 - 6 ounces firm tofu
2 large free-range eggs, lightly beaten
2 tbsp. nonfat grated cheddar cheese

1/4 cup scallions, chopped
Mrs. Dash or Spicy Mrs. Dash
1/8 - 1/4 tsp. paprika

1. Spray a 10-inch nonstick frying pan with enough spray to evenly coat it.
2. Heat the pan on a medium temperature, while crumbling the tofu into the pan.
3. As the tofu is cooking it dries slightly; then add the scallions and cook for about 3 minutes.
4. Add the lightly beaten eggs to this mixture and scramble until firm, adding the grated cheddar just before removing the pan from the heat.
5. Season to taste.

Makes 2 servings

High Protein Breakfast Shake

1 cup vanilla soy milk (Vita-Soy, Soy-um)
1 medium banana
4 large strawberries
1/2 cup nonfat yogurt, cottage cheese, ricotta cheese, or tofu.
1 tsp. - 1 tbsp. spirulina powder

1. Blend above ingredients together in blender.
2. If not sweet enough, add 1 tsp. pure maple syrup. Drink immediately.

Note: If made in a Vita-mix machine, the texture and blend are much smoother and finer, with greater emulsification.

Makes 1 serving

Notes:

French Toast

4 thick slices multi-grain bread
2 free-range eggs
1/2 cup vanilla soymilk
Pure maple syrup (optional)

Olive oil or canola oil-based spray
Molly McButter
Cinnamon / Sucanat

1. Beat together the eggs and soymilk.
2. Spray a nonstick frying pan or griddle with the oil-based spray just to thinly coat it.
3. Heat the skillet at a high heat until a drop of water sizzles when it hits the griddle.
4. Dip the slices of bread in the egg mixture, one at a time, to coat both sides evenly.
5. Cook on each side until the toast is golden brown, crispy on the outside and slightly soft on the inside when pressed with a spatula.
6. Lightly sprinkle with Molly McButter, cinnamon and sucanat, or a little maple syrup.

Makes 2 servings

Tropical Fruit Salad

1 papaya, diced
1 mango, diced
1 medium banana, sliced
1 cup pineapple, cubed
1 kiwi, sliced

1 medium orange, in sections
Juice of 1 lime
2 tbsp. unsweetened shredded coconut
2 tbsp. chopped dates or figs
Juice from prepared fresh fruit

Mix all ingredients together and serve immediately in your most elegant dishes.

Makes 4 servings

Notes:

Authentic Muesli

1 cup cold water	2 tbsp. dried fruit, finely chopped
1 cup old fashioned oatmeal	6 almonds, chopped or sliced
Juice of 1 small lemon	2 tbsp. sesame seeds
1 tbsp. wheatgerm	1 cup soymilk or plain, nonfat yogurt
2 tbsp. pure maple syrup	Cinnamon and Nutmeg, to taste
1 unpeeled apple, finely diced	Nutritional yeast, optional, but recommended
1 medium banana, sliced	

1. Combine the water and the oatmeal in a pyrex bowl. Let stand overnight, covered.
2. Add a little more water if the mixture seems too thick for your preference.
3. Just before serving, stir in rest of ingredients, except soymilk, spices and yeast.
4. Serve in individual bowls and allow each person to add the last 3 items to taste.

Makes 4 - 6 servings

Oatmeal Pancakes

1/2 cup whole wheat flour	1/4 cup applesauce
1/4 cup rolled oats	1/2 tsp. cinnamon
1 tsp. baking soda	Olive oil or canola oil-based spray
1 free-range egg	Molly McButter / Fruit preserves
3/4 cup buttermilk	Applesauce

1. Combine all of the dry ingredients, including the cinnamon, in a glass bowl.
2. Whip together all of the liquid ingredients in a blender.
3. Fold the liquid ingredients into the dry just until blended. Let sit for a few minutes.
4. Pour the pancake batter onto a hot, lightly sprayed, griddle or skillet.
5. When tiny bubbles which form on the pancakes begin to burst, turn the pancakes. This takes about 1 - 1½ minutes on each side.
6. Serve pancakes hot with Molly McButter and fruit preserves, or applesauce.

Makes 6 - 8 pancakes or 3 - 4 servings

Notes:

Potato and Egg Scramble

1/2 medium onion, chopped   2 leftover baked potatoes, diced
2 cloves of garlic, chopped   Mrs. Dash or Spicy Mr. Dash, to taste
2 free-range eggs, lightly beaten   Hot pepper sauce, to taste
4 ounces firm tofu, crumbled   Molly McButter, to taste

1.   Spray a medium skillet lightly with an olive oil or canola oil-based spray.
2.   Briefly saute the garlic and onion, for about 1 minute, at medium to high heat.
3.   Add diced potato and briefly saute for about 1 minute more.
4.   Add crumbled tofu and beaten eggs.
5.   Scramble until firm, adding seasoning just prior to completion of cooking.

Makes 2 servings

Scrambled Tofu and Tomatoes

1/2 medium onion, chopped   1/2 large green pepper, sliced
2 cloves fresh garlic, chopped   2 medium fresh tomatoes
6 ounces of firm tofu   Mrs. Dash or Spicy Mrs. Dash, to taste
                                    Cayenne pepper, to taste

1.   Lightly spray a medium skillet with an olive oil or canola oil-based spray.
2.   Briefly saute the garlic and onions, for about 1 minute, at medium to high heat.
3.   Crumble the tofu into the skillet. Add the green peppers and tomatoes.
4.   Saute the mixture, at medium heat, for about 2 - 3 minutes.
5.   Add seasoning to taste and serve.

Makes 2 servings

Notes:

Low Fat Banana Apricot Loaf

Though this is one item that may require more preparation time than most of the recipes in this book, once prepared you have several quick servings to look forward to. A slice makes an enjoyable breakfast food, a great snack or a special dessert with a flavored nonfat yogurt topping.

Dry ingredients:

1½ cups wholewheat flour
1/2 cup old fashioned oats
1/8 cup wheat germ
1½ tsp. non-aluminum based baking powder
1/2 tsp. baking soda
1 tsp. ground cinnamon
1/4 tsp. ground nutmeg
1/8 tsp. ground cloves
1/4 cup dried apricots, finely chopped

Moist ingredients:

2 free-range eggs
1/2 cup buttermilk
3 large or 4 medium bananas
1/2 cup dried prune puree*
   or applesauce
1/8 to 1/4 cup pure maple syrup

1.   Spray a nonstick or pyrex loaf pan with an olive oil or canola oil-based spray.
2.   In a large glass bowl, mix all of the dry ingredients, adding the apricots last.
3.   In a blender, whip all of the moist ingredients until very well blended.
4.   Fold the moist ingredients into the dry ingredients until just blended. Do not over mix, or tunnels will form in the finished baked product.
5.   Bake in a preheated 325° - 350° oven, for approximately one hour. Use a knitting needle or fork to test the middle of the loaf for doneness.

* Prune Puree: To prepare 1 cup of prune puree, combine 8 ounces (1 1/3 cups) of pitted prunes with 6 - 8 tbsp. of hot water in a Vita-Mix machine or food processor.

An alternative to preparing your own, is to buy a commercial product called **Just Like Shortenin'.** See the **Resources** section for information on where to find this product.

Notes: _____

Breakfast Bulgur

1 cup bulgur   1 cup fresh pineapple chunks
3 cups water   1 tbsp. pure maple syrup
2 tbsp. dried fruit, unsulphured   2 cups acidophilus milk or nonfat yogurt

1.   Bring water to a boil. Add the bulgur and return to a boil.
2.   Add the dried fruit and simmer the bulgur mixture for 10 minutes.
3.   Remove from the heat and add pineapple chunks and maple syrup.
4.   Let sit for 15 minutes and then serve.
5.   Top each serving with about 1/2 cup acidophilus milk or yogurt.

Makes 3 - 4 servings.

Brown Rice Delight

1 cup cooked brown rice   1 - 2 tsp. pure maple syrup or sucanat
1 cup fresh mango, chopped   1/2 cup plain, nonfat yogurt
2 tbsp. sesame tahini

Mix together all of the ingredients, and serve.

Variations: 1.   Substitute mango with other fresh, ripe fruit.
               2.   Substitute mango with a combination of pineapple, banana and mango.
               3.   Substitute tahini with 4 - 6 chopped almonds, and 1/4 tsp. almond extract.
               4.   Substitute mango with 2 tbsp. unsulphured dried fruit.

Makes 2 servings

Notes: _____

The Green Machine Shake

2 scoops Nature's Life Super-Green 1/2 cup plain, nonfat yogurt
   Pro-96 Powder   1 medium banana
1 tbsp. wheat germ*   1/2 cup strawberries, or other berries
1 tbsp. nutritional yeast*   1 tbsp. spirulina powder*
1 cup vanilla soymilk

In a blender or Vita-Mix machine, blend all ingredients together until smooth.

*If you have never used these items before, it is wise to start with about 1 tsp. each and gradually, over 3 - 4 weeks, build up to the recommended amounts in the recipe.

Makes 1 serving

Fruity Yogurt

2 cups plain nonfat yogurt w/acidophilus   1 medium banana sliced
1/2 cup blueberries   1 - 1½ tbsp. pure maple syrup
1 cup sliced strawberries   1/2 - 1 tsp. cinnamon

1. Blend yogurt, maple syrup and cinnamon together. Fold in all of the fruit.
2. Place in a covered container and let marinate in refrigerator for at least 4 hours, preferably overnight.
3. Serve, as is, in a parfait dish, or sprinkle no added fat granola over the top of the yogurt, for extra fiber.
4. Can use any fruits, in season, in place of above fruits.

Makes 4 servings

Notes:

Crazy Mixed-Up Grains

ONE:

2 cups mixed leftover grains
4 - 6 almonds, chopped

3 - 6 pieces soaked prunes and apricots*
1 - 2 tbsp. pure maple syrup or sucanat

Mix all ingredients together and serve with acidophilus milk or yogurt, and fruit sauce.

* See recipe on page 71 of this book.

Makes 2 servings

TWO:

1/4 cup raw millet
1/4 cup raw buckwheat groats
1/4 cup raw old fashioned oats
1/4 cup raw brown rice
1/2 inch fresh ginger root, peeled

2 - 2½ cups boiling water
1 - 2 tbsp. pure maple syrup or sucanat
4 - 6 almonds, chopped
3 - 6 pieces of soaked prunes and apricots
Nonfat acidophilus milk or plain, nonfat yogurt

1. Grind each of the grains and ginger root in a coffee mill, or a Vita-Mix machine. In a coffee mill, each will have to be ground separately to preserve the motor, and then mixed together. In a Vita-Mix, they can be ground together at the same time.
2. Add the boiling water to the ground grains and let sit for 30 minutes. Add as much water as necessary to get your desired consistency.
3. Add the maple syrup, fruit and almonds just prior to serving.
4. Top with acidophilus milk or yogurt and fruit sauce, e.g., Apple and Strawberry Sauce.

Makes 2 servings

Berrie Good Kasha

1 cup buckwheat groats
2 cups water
2 tbsp. unsulphured raisins
4 chopped dried apricots, unsulphured

1 tbsp. pure maple syrup
1 cup fresh berries
6 almonds, chopped
1/2 - 1 cup plain, nonfat yogurt

1. Bring the water to a boil. Add the groats and return to a boil.
2. Add the dried fruit, and simmer the mixture for 7 - 10 minutes.
3. When the groats are done, add the maple syrup, berries and almonds, and serve.
4. Top each serving with a generous portion of yogurt.

Makes 3 - 4 servings

Fruit Smoothies

Each recipe makes 2 servings

#1: Berrie Good

1 cup fresh berries

1 medium banana

1 cup pure organic apple cider

1 tbsp. spirulina powder

In a blender or Vita-Mix machine, blend all ingredients together until smooth.

#2: High Energy

1 cup plain, nonfat yogurt

1 fresh papaya

1 medium banana

1 tbsp. wheatgerm (build up to this)*#

1 tbsp. nutritional yeast (build up to this)*#

1 - 2 tsp. pure maple syrup or sucanat

1 tbsp. sesame seeds

1 tbsp. spirulina powder (build up to this)*#

In a blender or Vita-Mix machine, blend all ingredients together until smooth.

Variations: Add or substitute strawberries, blueberries, raspberries, mango, peaches, apricots, pineapple, pear, or other fresh, ripe fruit.

* If you have never used these products before (i.e., wheat germ, nutritional yeast, and spirulina powder), it is wise to start with about 1 tsp. each and gradually, over 3 - 4 weeks, build up to the recommended amounts in this recipe.

Any of these items can be added to any blended drink included in this book, as well as to sandwich fillings, or sprinkled on the top of salads, or mixed into loaves, burgers, or soups. They are so packed full of valuable nutrients, that it would be a shame to miss such easy opportunities to include them in your diet.

#3: Melon Ice

1 medium cantaloupe

1 - 2 tbsp. spirulina powder

4 - 6 ice cubes

In a blender or Vita-Mix machine, blend all ingredients together until smooth.

#4 : Ginger Snap

1 cup raspberries

4 fresh or dried, soaked apricots

1 cup fresh pineapple

1/2 inch fresh ginger root

In a blender or Vita-Mix machine, blend all ingredients together until smooth.

Variations:

1. Substitute the fruits in recipe **#4** with 1 papaya and 1 banana.

2. Substitute the fruits in recipe **#4** with 1 cup any berries, 1 banana, and 1 cup organic apple cider.

3. For **Plain, Nonfat Yogurt Fruit Smoothies**, add 1 cup of plain, nonfat yogurt to any of Smoothies listed above, except **#2: High Energy.** If the taste is too tart or too tangy, add 1 - 2 tsp. pure maple syrup or sucanat. Gradually reduce the sweetener each time you prepare the smoothie, until you no longer need it.

Notes: _____

Fruit Frappes

Make frappes in a blender or Vita-Mix machine, blending suggested fruits with 4 - 6 ice cubes. Try mixing your own blends of fruits. Serve immediately. Each combination makes 2 servings.

Variations:
1. **Pineapple and Mango Frappe**: 1 fresh ripe mango and 1 cup fresh pineapple plus ice.
2. **Raspberry and Banana Frappe**: 1 cup fresh or frozen raspberries and 1 ripe banana plus ice. Can use strawberries or blueberries instead.
3. **Mango and Papaya Frappe**: 1 ripe mango and 1 ripe papaya plus ice.
4. **Cantaloupe Frappe**: Pulp of 1 small cantaloupe plus ice.
5. **Banana and Papaya Frappe**: 1 ripe banana and 1 ripe papaya plus ice.
6. **Peach and Banana Frappe**: 1 ripe peach with skin and 1 ripe banana plus ice.
7. **Apple and Strawberry Frappe**: 1 cup pure organic apple cider and 1 cup fresh strawberries plus ice. Can substitute strawberries with pineapple, grapes, peach, papaya, banana, or pear.
8. **YOGURT FRAPPE:** Plain, **nonfat yogurt** can be added to any of the above combinations.

Note: If a sweeter taste is preferred, add 1 - 2 tsp. pure maple syrup or sucanat. However, the goal is to reduce your desire for sweets, so gradually reduce the amount of sweetener added each time you prepare the frappes.

Notes:

Fruit and Yogurt Whips and Puddings

The following recipes can be prepared in a blender or a Vita-Mix machine. The Vita-Mix machine produces a much finer and smoother consistency.

Chill each blend in the freezer for at least 1 hour before serving.

Each recipe makes 2 servings.

Fresh Nonfat Banana Yogurt

Blend 1 cup plain nonfat yogurt, 1 ripe banana and 2 tsp. pure maple syrup together. Add a drop of almond extract or a 1/2 tsp. of cinnamon or ginger for variety.

Variation: For **Tropical Fruit Yogurt**, substitute 1 cup of tropical fruits, eg. pineapple, mango, papaya, kiwi, banana, or avocado. It can be one of these or a combination.

                  Two methods: a) Blend ingredients together; or b) Mix chunks of fruit into plain, nonfat yogurt. For both methods, chill overnight to blend flavors.

Home-Blended Nonfat Vanilla Yogurt

Blend 1 cup plain, nonfat yogurt, 2 tsp. pure maple syrup, 1/4 - 1/2 tsp. pure vanilla extract. This combination can be the base for a variety of fruit and yogurt combinations.

Variation: 1.   For **Whipped Vanilla and Strawberry Yogurt**, add 1 cup fresh strawberries to the above ingredients and whip.

            2.   For **Sweet Potato and Raisin Yogurt Whip**, add 1 medium   unpeeled baked sweet potato, and 2 tbsp. unsulphured raisins to the   above basic combination and whip.

Notes: _____

Whipped Prunes and Almond Yogurt

Whip together 1 cup plain, nonfat yogurt, 1/4 - 1/2 tsp. almond extract, and 1/2 cup soaked unsulphured pitted prunes (drained).

Variations: 1.   For **Whipped Peaches and Almond Yogurt**, substitute 1 large ripe peach for the prunes, and add 1 tsp. sucanat.

2.   For **Pineapple Almond Whip**, substitute 1 cup fresh pineapple for the prunes, and 1 tsp. sucanat, if necessary.

3.   For **Apricot Dream**, substitute 1/2 cup soaked unsulphured apricots (drained) for the prunes, and add 4 - 5 raw almonds.

4.   For **Date and Almond Whip**, substitute 1/2 cup of soaked unsulphured dates (undrained) for the prunes, and add 6 raw almonds.

5.   For **Sweet Potato and Raisin Yogurt Whip**, substitute 1 medium unpeeled baked sweet potato, and 2 tbsp. unsulphured raisins for the prunes.

6.   For **Tofu-Yogurt Almond Pudding with Raspberry Puree**, add 1/2 cup soft tofu, 5 raw almonds and 2 tsp. sucanat. Top with Raspberry Puree (see **Blended Fruit Toppings** section).

Berry-Ricotta Surprise

In a blender or Vita-mix machine, blend 1 cup lowfat ricotta cheese with 1 cup of berries, (any one of, or a combination of, strawberries, raspberries, blueberries, blackberries), 1/4 - 1/2 tsp. brandy extract, 1/2 tsp. cinnamon, and 1 tbsp. pure maple syrup or sucanat. Chill in the freezer for at least 1 hour before serving.

Variation: 1.   For **Fruit-Ricotta Surprise**, substitute any fresh fruit in season for the berries. Peaches are particularly good. Use 2 medium peaches, unpeeled.

2.   For **Tropical Fruit-Ricotta Surprise**, substitute tropical fruits, eg. pineapple, kiwi, mango, papaya, or banana, or a combination of these. Add 1/2 tsp. dried ginger, or 1/2 inch fresh ginger, grated, to this blend.

Blended Fruit Toppings

Apple and Strawberry Sauce

1 fresh sweet unpeeled apple, cored   1/4 cup nonfat, plain yogurt
1 cup fresh strawberries   1/4 tsp. brandy extract

In a blender, or Vita-Mix machine, blend all ingredients until smooth. The consistency is much smoother with the latter.

Variations:

1. For **Banana and Pineapple Fruit Sauce / Topping**, substitute 1 ripe banana and 1 cup of fresh pineapple for the apple and strawberries.

2. For **Raspberry Puree**, substitute 2 cups of fresh raspberries for the apple and strawberries. Can eliminate the yogurt for a rich berry flavor.

3. For **Blueberry Sauce**, substitute 2 cups of blueberries for the fruit.

4. For **Tropical Fruit Sauce / Topping**, substitute 1 mango, 1 papaya and 1 cup fresh pineapple, for apple and strawberries.

5. For **Blended Fruit Topping**, use the Apple and Strawberry Sauce above, or substitute with any fruit or fruits you particularly like.

6. For **Apricot Sauce**, substitute 1 cup soaked unsulphured (drained) apricots for the apple and strawberries. Or substitute 1/2 cup apricots for only one of the fruits, creating **Apricot-Apple Sauce** or **Strawberry-Apricot Sauce**.

7. Substitute the strawberries with any other berries in season.

8. Substitute the brandy extract with almond, vanilla, lemon, orange, etc.

9. Substitute the apple and strawberries with any other fruits in season.

10. Substitute the fresh fruit with soaked dried fruits and some of the soaking liquid.

11. Add 1 - 2 tsp. pure maple syrup or sucanat, if desire a sweeter taste. The riper the fruit, the sweeter the sauce, naturally, without added sweetener.

12. For a **Non-Creamy Blended Fruit Topping**, prepare as above, but eliminate the yogurt.

Note: For information on how to soak dried fruit see the recipe for **Prunes and Apricots for Topping on Cereal**.

Frozen Fruits

Variations: 1.   For **Frozen Grapes**, remove seedless grapes from vines, wash thoroughly and dry. Put grapes into ziplock freezer bags, removing any air. Freeze grapes and eat as desired.

2.   For **Frozen Bananas**, use only ripe bananas with brown spots on the skin. Peel bananas and freeze in ziplock freezer bags. Slice and eat, or run them through the blender for a creamier consistency.

3.   For **Frozen Banana and Date Delight**, blend 1 frozen banana and 1/4 - 1/2 cup soaked unsulphured dates (drained) together. Refreeze before eating. For creamier consistency, run again through the blender just before serving. Makes 2 servings.

4.   For **Blended Frozen Bananas with Raisins**, blend 1 frozen banana and 2 tbsp. unsulphured raisins together. Can also add 1/4 tsp. almond extract to the blend.

5.   Freeze other fruits, eg. blueberries, peaches, pineapple, cantaloupe, mango, etc. Eat either as they are, or run them through the blender.

Note: When blending any of the above frozen fruit combinations, use "whip" speed on blender, or "high" speed on Vita-Mix machine. Refreeze after whipping and then serve. For a creamier blend, whip again very briefly, and serve.

Notes: _____

Beverages

Ginger Tea

1½ inches fresh ginger root, peeled
4 cups water
1 cup skimmed/lite evaporated milk, or vanilla soymilk
1 - 2 tsp. pure maple syrup

1. Bring water to a rolling boil. Add peeled ginger root.
2. Simmer ginger root in water for about 20 - 25 minutes.
3. Remove pot with ginger and water from heat.
4. Add evaporated milk, or soymilk, and maple syrup.
5. Can be served hot or iced.

Makes 3-4 servings.

Spiced Apple Cider

7 cups organic apple cider   1/4 tsp. nutmeg
3 cups orange juice, fresh squeezed 4 - 6 whole cloves
4 - 6 cinnamon sticks   1 large unpeeled orange, thinly sliced

1. Combine all ingredients in a Dutch oven or stock pot.
2. Heat just to boiling. Cover and keep hot on very low heat.
3. Ladle servings as desired. Include a slice of orange on the surface of each.

Notes: _____

Soups

<u>Split Pea Soup</u>

1 lb. dried green split peas
8 cups hot water
4 large carrots, chopped
4 large stalks celery, chopped
1 medium onion, chopped
2 large cloves of garlic, minced
1 tbsp. pure virgin olive oil (optional)

1/2 tsp. Real Salt
1 tsp. Spicy Mrs. Dash
1/4 tsp. fresh ground pepper
1/2 tsp. dried basil
1/4 tsp. ground cumin
1/2 tsp. dried marjoram
Juice of 1 fresh lemon
Hot pepper sauce, to taste

1. Sort and wash peas. Place in a Dutch oven with the hot water.
2. Add the remaining ingredients, except the lemon juice and hot pepper sauce.
3. Bring to a boil, and then simmer for about 1½ hours, until the peas are soft and the vegetables are tender.
4. When the soup is finished cooking, add the juice of the lemon, and the hot pepper sauce. Let the soup sit for about 15 minutes before serving to allow the flavors to develop.

Variation: To create a **Mediterranean Lentil Soup**, add 1 carton (26 ounces) of Pomi tomatoes, 1 medium green pepper, chopped, and 1/2 inch fresh ginger, grated, with the rest of the ingredients, at the start of cooking. Then add 3 medium zucchini, sliced, 10 minutes before cooking is complete. As in Step #4 above, add lemon juice and hot pepper sauce, and let sit 15 minutes before serving.

Note: This soup tastes even better the next day. But don't bring it to a boil again after the lemon juice and hot pepper sauce have been added! It will develop a slightly bitter after taste.

Makes 6 - 8 servings

Notes: _____

Minestrone Soup

1 medium onion, chopped
2 large cloves of garlic, minced
4 cups hot water
2 large carrots, chopped
1 large stalk of celery, chopped
1 carton (26 ounces) Pomi tomatoes
1/4 cup fresh parsley, chopped
3 medium unpeeled potatoes, chopped
1 tsp. dried basil
1 tbsp. Spicy Mrs. Dash

1/2 cup whole grain macaroni
2 small zucchini, chopped
1 cup kale, chopped
1 cup spinach, chopped
1/2 cup green cabbage, shredded
1 can (16 ounces) kidney beans,
        drained and rinsed
1/4 - 1/2 tsp. hot pepper sauce (optional)
Parmesan or Romano cheese

1. In a Dutch oven, bring the 4 cups of water to a boil. Add all of the ingredients in the first column and return to a boil.
2. Cover and simmer for about 20 minutes.
3. Add the rest of the ingredients, except the hot pepper sauce, and simmer for another 25 minutes. More water can be added as necessary, if the soup becomes too thick.
4. Add hot pepper sauce when cooking is complete, and let marinate for about 10 minutes before serving.
5. Top each serving with a sprinkling of Parmesan or Romano cheese.

Makes 6 - 8 servings

Curried Lentil Soup

1 lb. lentils
10 cups of water
1 large onion, chopped
3 medium cloves of garlic, minced
2 large carrots, sliced
1 large stalk of celery, chopped
3 large unpeeled potatoes, chopped

2 - 3 tsp. curry powder
1/4 cup fresh parsley, chopped
1/2 inch fresh ginger root, grated
1 - 2 tsp. Spicy Mrs. Dash
1/4 tsp. fresh ground pepper
Plain, nonfat yogurt

1. Put all of the ingredients, except the yogurt, into a Dutch oven. Bring to a boil.
2. Cover and simmer for 1 hour, until lentils are tender.
3. Top each serving with a dollop of yogurt.

Makes 8 - 10 servings.

Miso Soup with Tofu Cubes

4 cups of water
4 pieces, 1 inch each, of wakame
       seaweed, dried
1/2 cup of water
1/2 cup carrots, thinly sliced

1/2 cup daikon radish, thinly sliced
4 mushrooms, quartered
4 ounces firm tofu, cubed
4 tbsp. red or barley miso
2 scallions, finely sliced

1. Reconstitute the wakame in 1/2 cup of water.
2. Bring 4 cups water to a boil. Add carrot and daikon and cook for 2 minutes.
3. Add mushrooms and cook for another 3 minutes.
4. Reduce to medium heat and add tofu cubes. Water should not boil after tofu is added. (Tofu will become hard if it is boiled.)
5. Add wakame and soaking water, when tofu floats to the surface. Do not boil water!
6. Remove 1/3 - 1/2 cup of water from the pot and use to cream the miso. Only when the paste has been fully dissolved, is it returned to the pot. Do not boil the soup!
7. After soup is removed from the heat, sprinkle with scallions and serve.

Makes 4 servings.

Instant Miso Soup

Boil 1 cup of water. Pour a small amount of the water into a cup. Cream 1 tbsp. of red or barley miso in this water, and then pour the rest of the water into the cup. Mix, and then top with tiny tofu pieces and finely chopped scallions. *A healthy mid-afternoon pickup!*

Notes:

Lentil Vegetable Soup

1 lb. lentils
10 cups water
1 large onion, chopped
2 large cloves of garlic, minced
2 large carrots, sliced
2 large stalks celery, chopped
1 small green pepper, chopped
1 carton (26 ounces) Pomi tomatoes
1 lb. fresh spinach, chopped

1/4 cup fresh parsley, chopped
1/2 tsp. dried oregano
1/2 tsp. ground cumin
1 bay leaf
1/2 tsp. dried red pepper
1/4 tsp. fresh ground pepper
1 tsp. Mrs. Dash
Juice of one lemon

1. Put all of the ingredients, except lemon juice, into a Dutch oven, and bring to a boil.
2. Cover and simmer for about 1 hour, until the lentils are tender, stirring occasionally.
3. Add lemon juice when cooking is complete, and let the pot sit off the heat, covered, for 15 minutes, before serving.

Variations: 1. For **Potato and Lentil Soup**, add 4 unpeeled, chopped potatoes to the Dutch oven, with the rest of the ingredients, and cook for 1 hour as above. Add lemon juice at end of cooking and let sit before serving.

2. For another version of **Potato and Lentil Soup**, eliminate the carton of tomatoes and the spinach, and add 6 unpeeled, chopped potatoes. The lemon juice is optional with this variation.

Note: This soup tastes even better the next day. But don't boil it the next day when you are reheating it, as this can result in a bitter aftertaste.

Makes 8 - 10 servings

Notes:

Sandwiches

Chicken Pita Sandwich

1½ cups skinless chicken breast
  cooked and diced
1 stalk of celery, diced
1/2 green pepper, diced
1/2 cup unwaxed cucumber, diced
4 scallions, diced
Juice of 1/2 fresh lemon

2 tbsp. Nayonnaise
1/4 cup plain, nonfat yogurt
1 tbsp. Dijon mustard
1/8 tsp. Tabasco sauce
2 large pitas, wholewheat, in halves
alfalfa sprouts

Mix all of the ingredients together except the pitas and the sprouts. Fill each of 4 pockets with the filling and top each with alfalfa sprouts.

Variations:
1. Substitute the Dijon mustard with 1 - 2 tsp. curry powder.

2. For **Tuna Salad Sandwiches**, substitute the chicken with 1 can (6.5 ounces) water-packed, drained and rinsed tuna. Use 8 slices of whole grain bread, or 4 large whole grain rolls.

3. Fresh green leaf lettuce and slices of tomato can be used on each sandwich, or stuffed into the pita pockets.

Turkey Loaf on Wholewheat Kaiser Roll

See recipe in **Main Entrees** section for Turkey Loaf.
Spread Dijon mustard or Nayonnaise, or a combination of both on the Roll.
Slices of each of, a red onion, and a ripe tomato, add a flavorful accent.

Wholewheat English Muffin Pizzas

1. Spread some bottled nonfat natural marinara sauce onto 2 halves of an English muffin.

2. Sprinkle a little bottled minced garlic and some diced scallions over the sauce.

3. Arrange slices of fresh mushrooms, and some grated nonfat cheddar or mozzarella cheese on top.

4. Sprinkle with Parmesan cheese and fresh ground pepper.

5. Bake, on a lightly sprayed cookie sheet, at 450º, until cheeses are melted.

Marinated Tofu and Sprout Sandwich

1. Slice an 8 ounce block of extra firm tofu into 1/4 to 1/2 inch thick slices.
2. Place the slices side by side in a shallow pyrex baking dish.
3. Cover the slices with a marinade of your choice (see **Marinades** section). Be adventurous and try a different one each time you do it.
4. Then cover the dish and refrigerate for at least 4 hours, preferably overnight.
5. When ready to serve, simply place several slices of marinated tofu on a slice of whole grain bread, add some fresh tomato slices and a generous portion of alfalfa sprouts.

So you're in a hurry? You have no time to marinate tofu, but that's what you want to eat. Place a few slices of tofu on a flat plate and pour some Bragg's Liquid Aminos over them, followed by some fresh squeezed lemon or lime juice. Wait about 5 minutes, and there you have it! Marinated tofu in a flash!

Variation: 1.   For a **Marinated Tempeh Sandwich,** substitute the tofu slices with any of the many varieties and flavors of tempeh.

                2.   A **Tempeh Sandwich** does not have to start with marinated tempeh. Tempeh comes in many flavors which are very tasty as they are. Dress this sandwich as suggested for the marinated tofu sandwich. You could also add a touch of Dijon mustard or Nayonnaise.

Notes:

Turkey Burger, American Style

1 lb. ground turkey breast
1/2 medium onion, diced
1 stalk of celery, diced
1/2 green pepper, diced
2 cloves of garlic, minced

1 tsp. paprika
1/4 tsp. fresh ground pepper
1 tbsp. Bragg's Liquid Aminos
4 whole wheat burger buns
Dijon mustard, lettuce, tomatoes

1.   Combine the ground turkey and the seasonings.
2.   Shape the mixture into 4 patties.
3.   Grill, or pan fry in a nonstick skillet until cooked throughout, about 5 minutes per side.

Variations: Dress your burger with a variety of toppings such as:

cucumber slices	radishes	sliced mushrooms
alfalfa or clover sprouts	chutneys	chunky salsa
nonfat chili beans	onion slices	tomato slices
Nayonnaise	Dijon mustard	shredded lettuce
grated nonfat cheese	Gourmet mustards	

Turkey Burger, Asian Style

1 lb. ground turkey breast
1/2 medium onion, diced
1 tbsp. soy sauce, reduced sodium
2 cloves of garlic, minced

1/2 inch fresh ginger root, grated
1½ tsp. sesame oil
1/4 tsp. dry mustard powder

1.   Thoroughly combine all of the ingredients.
2.   Shape the mixture into 4 patties.
3.   Grill, or pan fry in a nonstick skillet until cooked throughout, about 5 minutes each side.
4.   See Variations above for ways to dress your burger.

Notes:

Eggless "Egg" Salad Sandwich

1/2 lb. firm tofu	1 tbsp. tahini
1 medium carrot, shredded	1 tbsp. Dijon mustard
2 scallions, finely chopped	1 tsp. Spicy Mrs. Dash
1/4 cup fresh parsley, chopped	1/4 tsp. fresh ground pepper

1. Mash the drained tofu with a fork to form very loose curds.
2. Combine thoroughly with the rest of the ingredients.
3. Spread on wholegrain bread, toast or crackers. Also great with lowfat tortilla chips, or with vegetables, as a **Tofu Vegetable Dip.**

Note: This product is best used immediately. It does not store well.

Notes:

Nonfat Cheese and Avocado Pita Pocket with Sprouts

1. Into a whole wheat pita pocket, put strips of fresh, ripe avocado; about 1/4 of a medium avocado.

2. Sprinkle 1 ounce of grated nonfat cheese over the avocado.

3. Stuff the pocket with chunky salsa and clover or alfalfa sprouts.

4. Pour **Tahini and Buttermilk Dressing** (see **Salad Dressings** section) over the filling in the pocket.

Turkey and Tomato on Rye

1. On 100% rye bread, spread a combination of 1 tsp. Nayonnaise and 1 tsp. Dijon or grain mustard.

2. Place 2 ounces of thinly sliced turkey breast on the spread.

3. Dress with green leaf lettuce, and cucumber and tomato slices.

4. Top with another slice of wholesome rye bread.

Almond Butter, Tomato and Sprouts on Multigrain Bread

Though a bit high in fat, this sandwich is packed full of nutrition!

Go easy on the almond butter; no more than 2 tbsp. The rest is self-explanatory. Other veggies that go well with almond butter include cucumber slices, green pepper rings, onions, avocado (Cut the almond butter down to 1 tbsp. if you use 1/4 of an avocado.), fruit preserves, dried fruits, chunky salsa and radish slices.

Note: Always buy fresh ground, natural almond butter out of a refrigerated case instead of taking it from a shelf, as it tends to go rancid quickly in warmer temperatures. And due to being ground, there is more surface area of the product exposed to the oxygen in the air, which is the reason for rancidity occurring in the first place.

Bean Burritos with Salsa and Yogurt

One of the quickest meals I know!

1.   Spoon some black beans (come in 16 ounce cans), slightly off center, onto a corn or whole wheat tortilla.

2.   Sprinkle some grated nonfat cheese over the beans, and a spoonful each of chunky salsa, and of plain, nonfat yogurt.

3.   Fold the short sides of the tortilla over the filling. Then fold over the long sides, placing the seam side down on the plate.

4.   They taste best when served warm. Serve with a salad of greens and tomatoes.

Salmon Dill Sandwich on Sprouted Bread

1/2 cup plain, nonfat yogurt
2 tbsp. Nayonnaise
2 scallions, finely chopped
1 tsp. dried dill weed
1 clove of garlic, minced

1/8 - 1/4 tsp. hot pepper sauce
Mrs. Dash, to taste
1 stalk of celery, diced
1 can (7.5 ounces) water-packed salmon,
    drained and rinsed

1.   Blend all of the seasoning ingredients together well.
2.   Add the salmon and celery, and combine thoroughly with the blended seasoning sauce.
3.   Cover and refrigerate for at least 1 hour.
4.   Prepare sandwiches on sprouted wholegrain bread. Delicious with alfalfa sprouts, tomato slices, and green or red leafy lettuces.

Notes:

Salads

Fresh Organic Salad Mix

Available, as is, ready to use, from various sources: farms which produce organic produce for wholesale and for mail order (see **Resources** section), health food stores, farmers' markets, and more recently, produce sections of many grocery stores.

Tossed Green Salad / Mixed Green Salad

You can use the organic salad mix, or mix your own variety of green, leafy vegetables. Look for the darkest green leaves, or the brightest red leaves. *Iceberg lettuce is not, by itself, a tossed green salad, as most restaurants would have you believe.* Some greens for you to explore, include:

arugula	endive	red cabbage
bibb lettuce	escarole	rocket
chicory	green cabbage	romaine
Chinese cabbage	head lettuce (Ithaca)	Savoy cabbage
collard greens	kale	spinach
corn salad (lamb's lettuce)	leaf lettuce (Buttercrunch)	Swiss chard
	parsley	watercress

Greens and Tomatoes

Mix about 3 different green (or red) leafy vegetables together and top with your favorite, in-season tomatoes, in chunks or slices, and your favorite dressing.

Spinach and Mushroom Salad / Spinach and Tomato Salad

Mix any variety of spinach (some examples are leaf or spring spinach, Malabar spinach, and New Zealand spinach) with sliced brown or white mushrooms and/or tomatoes. Dressings with a lemon, lime or mustard base make a tasty accent.

Romaine, Watercress and Tomato Salad

1 head of romaine lettuce   3 - 5 radishes, sliced
2 cups watercress leaves   1 large tomato, in chunks
2 scallions, finely chopped

1. Tear the romaine leaves into bite-size pieces.
2. Snip the watercress leaves into manageable pieces, with kitchen shears.
3. Toss all of the ingredients together and drizzle your favorite dressing over the salad.

Variation: For **Romaine and Tomato Salad**, eliminate the watercress. Then give this salad a real kick with a watercress dressing. (See **Salad Dressings**)

Makes 4 servings.

Notes: _____

Cucumber and Tomato Raita

2 cups plain, nonfat yogurt	1 medium onion, thinly sliced
2 - 3 large cloves of garlic, minced	1 large fresh, unwaxed cucumber
2 tbsp. fresh mint, chopped	2 large fresh tomatoes
1 - 2 tsp. Spicy Mrs. Dash	1/8 - 1/4 tsp. hot pepper sauce (optional)

1. Blend the yogurt, garlic and seasonings together. Set aside.
2. Dice the unpeeled cucumber and let it drain on paper towels.
3. Dice the tomatoes, and prepare the onions. Then combine the cucumbers, onions and tomatoes with the yogurt mixture.
4. Chill thoroughly, allowing at least 1 - 2 hours for the flavors to marinate and blend.

Variation: For **Zucchini Salad**, substitute the cucumber with 3 medium zucchini. For another version of **Zucchini Salad**, substitute the cucumber with the zucchini, eliminate the yogurt mixture, and top with the **Spicy Dressing**.

Note: This is a delicious side dish with spicy entrees, and with East Indian and Middle Eastern menus.

Makes 4 - 6 servings.

Red and Green Cabbage Slaw / Creamy Cabbage Slaw

1 medium head of red cabbage	1/3 cup plain, nonfat yogurt
1 medium head of green cabbage	1/4 cup organic cider vinegar
2 large carrots, shredded	1 tbsp. pure maple syrup
1 medium onion, chopped	1/4 tsp. celery seeds
1 large yellow pepper, in thin strips	1/4 to 1/2 tsp. hot pepper sauce
1/3 cup Nayonnaise	

1   Blend the Nayonnaise, yogurt, vinegar, syrup, seeds and hot pepper sauce together.
2. Thinly slice the red and green cabbages.
3. Toss all of the vegetables together in a large bowl.
4. Pour the dressing over the vegetables and toss well to combine. Chill thoroughly.

Makes 8 - 10 servings.

Lowfat Creamy Coleslaw

1 large head of green cabbage, sliced
1 medium onion, chopped
2 large carrots, shredded
3 tbsp. Nayonnaise
1/2 cup plain, nonfat yogurt

1/4 cup balsamic vinegar
Juice of 1 fresh lemon
1 tbsp. Bragg's Liquid Aminos
1/2 tsp. fresh ground pepper
1 tbsp. pure maple syrup

1. Blend everything, but the vegetables together. Let sit.
2. In a large bowl, toss the vegetables together.
3. Pour the dressing over the vegetables and toss well to combine. Chill thoroughly.

Variation: For **Nippy Dijon Coleslaw**, eliminate the lemon juice and maple syrup. Reduce the Bragg's liquid Aminos to 1 tsp. and add 2 tbsp. Dijon mustard, 1/4 to 1/2 tsp. dry mustard powder, 1/8 tsp. celery seeds and 1 tbsp. tahini.

Makes 6 - 8 servings.

Marinated Tomato, Onion and Cucumber Slices

Marinate the vegetables in a vinaigrette or herb dressing for 30 - 60 minutes. (See **Salad Dressings** section.) Cover and refrigerate while marinating.

Notes:

Three-Bean Salad

1/4 cup red wine vinegar
2 tbsp. organic cider vinegar
1 tbsp. pure virgin olive oil
2 medium cloves of garlic, minced
1/4 - 1/2 tsp. cayenne pepper
1 tbsp. pure maple syrup
1/2 tsp. dry mustard powder

1/2 medium red onion, sliced
2 large stalks of celery, chopped
2 cans (16 ounces each) red kidney
   beans, drained and rinsed
1 can (16 ounces) chickpeas, drained
   and rinsed
1 lb. fresh green beans, lightly cooked

1.   Combine all of the ingredients in the first column, in a large bowl.
2.   Add the onions, celery and beans, and toss gently. Cover and refrigerate.

Note: Make this salad the day before to allow the flavors to blend. Though it must be kept
       refrigerated when made ahead, this salad is best served at room temperature for fullest
       flavor.

Makes 8 - 10 servings.

Caesar Salad

Tear the leaves of 1 large head of romaine lettuce into large bite-size pieces. Toss gently, but
thoroughly, with the Caesar Dressing in the Dressings section.   Top with nonfat seasoned
croutons, available at most health food stores.

Variations: 1.   For a **Chicken Caesar** or a **Fish Caesar**, top the salad with pieces of
                   grilled chicken or fish, or canned tuna.

              2.   Make a **Seafood Caesar** by topping with a mixture of grilled shrimp,
                   scallops, crabmeat (or imitation crabmeat), lobster and whitefish.

              3.   Sprinkle 2 tbsp. of grated nonfat cheese and a few sesame seeds on top.

Notes: _____

Broccoli-Cauliflower Salad

1/4 cup buttermilk
1/4 cup Nayonnaise
2 tbsp. plain, nonfat yogurt
1 tbsp. sucanat
1/4 tsp. fresh ground pepper
Juice of 1 fresh lemon or lime

2 cups broccoli florets, small
2 cups cauliflower florets, small
2 scallions, chopped
1/2 large red pepper, chopped
1/2 small red onion, chopped
Hot pepper sauce (optional)

1. Blend all of the ingredients together in the first column.
2. In a large bowl, combine all of the vegetables in the second column.
3. Pour the dressing over the vegetables and toss lightly. Store in the refrigerator.

Note: For added flavor and nutrition, a handful of seeds, such as sesame, pumpkin or sunflower, can be sprinkled on top just prior to serving.

Makes 4 - 6 servings.

Creamy Potato Salad

3/4 cup plain, nonfat yogurt
1/4 cup Nayonnaise
1/4 cup organic cider vinegar
2 medium cloves of garlic, minced
1 tsp. Mrs. Dash or Spicy Mrs. Dash
1/2 - 1 tsp. dry mustard powder
1 tsp. curry powder
1/2 tsp. fresh ground pepper
Hot pepper sauce, to taste (optional)

8 medium potatoes, baked with skin
1/2 large red onion, chopped
2 large celery stalks, chopped
5 radishes, sliced
2 free-range hard-boiled eggs,
    sliced (optional)

1. In a large bowl, thoroughly combine all of the ingredients in the first column.
2. Chop the unpeeled potatoes into small bite-size pieces, and add to the bowl.
3. Add the remaining ingredients in the second column, except eggs, and toss gently.
4. Top the salad with the egg slices. Cover and refrigerate for at least 30 to 60 minutes.

Makes 8 servings.

Mediterranean Potato Salad

1 tbsp. pure virgin olive oil
Juice of 1 fresh lemon
1/4 cup balsamic vinegar
1/2 medium ripe avocado
1/2 cup plain, nonfat yogurt
2 medium cloves of garlic, minced
1 tsp. dried tarragon
1/4 tsp. fresh ground pepper
1 tsp. Spicy Mrs. Dash

6 medium potatoes, baked
1 large stalk celery, chopped
4 scallions, chopped
1/2 large green pepper, chopped
1 large tomato, chopped
10-15 black olives, chopped

1. In a large bowl, blend all of the ingredients in the first column thoroughly.
2. Chop the unpeeled potatoes into small bite-size pieces, and add to the bowl.
3. Add the remaining ingredients in the second column, and toss gently.
4. Cover and refrigerate for at least 30 to 60 minutes before serving.

Makes 6 - 8 servings.

Tri-Color Pasta and Vegetable Salad

1 package (16 ounces) fresh vegetable
    pasta: 3 colors in one package
1 can (16 ounces) black beans,
    drained and rinsed
2 medium zucchini, thickly sliced
1/2 lb. fresh broccoli, cauliflower or
    baby carrots, chopped
1 red, and 1 green pepper, chopped
3 scallions, chopped
1/4 cup fresh cilantro, chopped

1 cup plain, nonfat yogurt
1 cup chunky fresh salsa, medium
3 medium cloves of garlic, minced
1/2 tsp. ground cumin
1/2 tsp. fresh ground pepper
Juice of 1 fresh lime
Parmesan or Romano cheese, for
topping as desired

1. Combine all of the ingredients in the second column, except the cheese.
2. Cook the pasta according to the directions on the package.
3. Combine the cooked pasta, vegetables and dressing. Bake at 325 degrees for 30 minutes in a lightly sprayed casserole dish. *(The vegetables should not be soft.)*

Variations: 1.   Instead of heating this salad, serve it as a cold salad. As above, combine the cooked pasta, raw vegetables, and dressing. Chill thoroughly before serving. Sprinkle with Parmesan or Romano.

2.   Substitute any vegetables in season you desire for the carrots, broccoli or cauliflower, or use a combination of fresh vegetables.

3.   Grated nonfat cheddar or mozzarella cheese can be used instead of Parmesan or Romano.

4.   To make a **Tuna, Salmon or Crab Pasta Salad**, simply replace the beans in the recipe with a 6 ounce can of tuna or salmon, or 6 - 8 ounces of flaked crabmeat or the imitation variety. Serve hot or cold.

Notes: 1.   For **Pasta Salad**, see the above variations listed. Instead of using the tri-color variety of pasta, experiment with any wholegrain or vegetable pasta that appeals to you. Eat it cold or hot. The choice is yours!

2.   A quick and easy **Pasta and Vegetable Salad**, for those sudden potluck invitations or a very hurried dinner, can be made by cooking a batch of pasta and a batch of frozen vegetables (the Mediterranean variety is delicious!). And then tossing them together with any salad dressing of your choice. (See **Salad Dressings**) Or just use the dressing from the above recipe.

Makes 6 - 8 servings.

Notes:

Lively Chef's Salad

1 head dark green or red lettuce	6 cherry tomatoes, in halves
6 mushrooms, sliced	chickpeas
1/2 large green pepper, in thin strips	kidney beans
3 scallions, chopped	marinated cubes of tempeh or tofu
2 medium cloves of garlic, minced	Parmesan or Romano cheese

Dressing of your choice (see **Salad Dressings**)

1.   In a large bowl, combine all of the ingredients in the first column, and toss lightly.
2.   Add the cherry tomatoes and toss very gently, just to distribute them.
3.   Top each serving of salad with a spoonful of each of the beans, and a few cubes of tempeh or tofu. Sprinkle about 1 tbsp. of cheese onto each serving as well.

Variations: 1.   Leftover pieces of chicken or fish can be used instead of the beans.

2.   Grated nonfat cheese can be used in place of Parmesan or Romano.

3.   The basic salad, without the beans and tempeh, can be used as a side salad for another meal.

Note: To make **Marinated Tempeh**, or **Marinated Tofu**, simply slice the tempeh or the extra firm tofu into 1/4 - 1/2 inch thick slices, and place these slices side by side in a shallow pyrex dish. Cover the slices with a marinade of your choice (see **Marinades**). Then cover the dish and refrigerate for at least 4 hours, preferably overnight, if possible. When ready to serve, cut the slices into the size of cubes you desire. Whatever you do not use can be kept, covered, in the refrigerator, for up to 5 days, and used as desired.

Makes 4 servings.

Notes: _____

Imitation Crabmeat Salad

1 lb. imitation crabmeat, chopped	2 large tomatoes, chopped
1 tbsp. pure virgin olive oil	1 medium red pepper, chopped
2 medium cloves of garlic, minced	1 medium green pepper, diced
Juice of 2 - 3 fresh limes (1/2 cup juice)	2 tbsp. fresh cilantro, chopped
1 tsp. Mrs. Dash or Spicy Mrs. Dash	1/8 - 1/4 tsp. hot pepper sauce
1/2 tsp. red pepper flakes	
1 small red onion, diced	

1.   Combine all of the seasonings. Let sit while you chop the vegetables and meat.
2.   Add the chopped vegetables, cilantro and crabmeat to the sauce.
3.   Cover and refrigerate for at least 1 hour prior to serving. Keeps up to 3 days in the refrigerator.

Variations: 1.   Instead of imitation crabmeat, any variety of cooked white fish or seafood can be used.

2.   For **Bay Scallop Salad**, just substitute 1 lb. of bay scallops for the crabmeat.   Scallops are especially good prepared with this recipe.

3.   For a **Creamy Imitation Crabmeat Salad** to serve over a baked potato or grains, reduce the amount of lime juice to that of 1 fresh lime and add 1/2 cup plain, nonfat yogurt. Refrigerate for at least 1 hour.

Makes 4 servings.

Notes:

Citrus Rice and Bean Salad

2 cups brown rice, cooked
3 scallions, finely chopped
1 can (16 ounces) black beans,
    drained and rinsed
1 can (6 ounces) water-packed tuna
    or salmon, drained and rinsed
1 large orange, seedless, peeled and chopped

1/2 cup orange juice, fresh squeezed
2 tbsp. fresh cilantro, chopped
1 tbsp. pure virgin olive oil
1/4 cup nonfat, plain yogurt
2 tbsp. coarse grain mustard or
   Dijon mustard

1. In a Vita-Mix machine or blender combine all of the ingredients in the second column. Refrigerate until ready to use. Can be made ahead.
2. In a large bowl, combine all of the ingredients in the first column.
3. Pour the prepared dressing over the rice combination, and toss until well mixed.
4. Refrigerate until ready to serve.

Variations:

1. Substitute the tuna or salmon with 6 - 8 ounces (about 1 cup) of diced skinless chicken or turkey breast.

2. Substitute the tuna or salmon with **Marinated Tofu or Tempeh.** (See recipe under **Sandwich Fillings** or under **Lively Chef's Salad.**)

3. For a unique flavor, substitute the fresh squeezed orange juice in the dressing, with the juice of 1 - 2 fresh limes.

Makes 6 servings.

Kitchen Sink Salad

This is basically what it sounds like! Anything you need to use up is perfect for this salad. As long as it is fresh, natural and organic, throw it in. Include some leafy greens, a few other veggies, a little protein (tofu, legumes, fish or chicken), and top it off with some colorful fresh tomatoes. Select one of your favorite lowfat or nonfat dressings and *enjoy to your heart's content, your body's content, and your mind's content!!*

Curried Brown Rice Salad

6 cups cooked brown rice
4 cups cooked chicken or turkey
    breast, diced
2 large stalks of celery, chopped
1 small green pepper, chopped
1 small red pepper, chopped
1 can (16 ounces) chickpeas, drained
    and rinsed
1 cup fresh pineapple chunks
1 small red onion, diced

1 cup plain, nonfat yogurt
1/3 cup balsamic vinegar
3 medium cloves of garlic, minced
2 tsp. sesame oil
1 tbsp. Bragg's Liquid Aminos
2 tbsp. sucanat
2 tsp. curry powder
1 tsp. dry mustard powder
1 tsp. Mrs. Dash
1/4 tsp. fresh ground pepper

1. In a blender, thoroughly mix all of the dressing ingredients in the second column. Cover and refrigerate until ready to use.
2. In a large bowl, combine all of the salad ingredients in the first column.
3. Pour chilled dressing over the salad combination. Toss gently.
4. Cover and refrigerate for at least 30 minutes to blend the flavors.

Variations:

1. Substitute the chicken or turkey with equal portions of chopped fish, or shellfish, or imitation crabmeat, or a combination of scallops, shrimp, and whitefish.

2. Eliminate chicken or turkey, and add 1 cup of fresh green peas.

3. Substitute the poultry with marinated tofu or tempeh slices or cubes. Double the dressing recipe above and marinate the tofu or tempeh slices in this mixture, overnight, prior to use.

4. For **Curried Brown Rice, Salmon and Vegetable Salad**, substitute the chicken or turkey with 1 can (15 ounces) water-packed salmon, drained and rinsed, or 3 cups diced fresh baked salmon. Substitute the chickpeas with 1 can (16 ounces) of black-eyed peas. And add 1 cup of finely chopped raw broccoli and/or raw cauliflower.

Makes 8 - 10 servings.

Notes: _____

So What's in a Salad Bar?

The following is a set of lists to help you develop your own repertoire of salad bar ingredients! Be creative. Select different items from time to time, for interest and variety. Widen your scope of experience with respect to flavor and color combinations.

Start with the Greens: Each week select a few of these to include in your own potential salad bar.

Alfalfa sprouts
Amaranth
Beet tops
Bibb lettuce
Cabbage, red and green
Celery tops
Chicory
Chinese cabbage
Clover sprouts
Collards
Corn salad
Dandelion greens
Endive
Escarole
Head Lettuce

Kale
Lambsquarter
Mint
Parsley
Red or Green leaf lettuce
Rocket
Romaine lettuce
Spinach
Swiss Chard
Watercress

Then add Some Variety in Colors and Textures with more dense salad items. Use in smaller quantities.

Artichoke hearts, in water
Asparagus
Beets, raw, grated, or cooked
Bell peppers
Broccoli, raw or lightly steamed
Carrots, shredded, sliced, steamed
Cauliflower, raw or lightly steamed
Celery
Chives
Corn
Cucumbers
Green beans
Jicama
Legumes: chickpeas, black-eyed peas
         black beans, kidney beans

Mushrooms, brown and white
Okra
Onions, red and white, Bermuda
Pickles, low sodium
Potatoes, cooked
Radishes, red and daikon
Scallions
Snow peas
Sprouts, any variety
Squash, winter, summer, zucchini
Tomatoes, any variety
Sweet peas
Sweet potatoes

And Then Complete the Makings of a Great Salad, before you dress it!

Avocados, fresh and ripe (Go easy!)
Bread, wholegrain varieties
Brown rice, cooked
Buckwheat groats, cooked
Bulgur wheat, cooked
Cheese, nonfat or lowfat
Chicken, skinless breast, cooked
Crackers, wholegrain, nonfat
Croutons, wholegrain, nonfat
Eggs, free-range, hard boiled
Fish, cooked
Herbs and Spices
Kasha, cooked

Marinated beans, nonfat or lowfat
Millet, cooked
Olives, black or green (Go easy!)
Nuts, esp. almonds (Go very easy!)
Pasta, wholegrain or vegetable, cooked

Poppy seeds
Pumpkin seeds
Raisins
Salmon, canned, water-packed
Sesame seeds and Tahini (Go Easy!)
Sunflower seeds
Shellfish, cooked
Tempeh, as is, or marinated
Tofu, as is, or marinated
Tuna, canned, water-packed
Turkey, skinless breast, cooked

The Grand Finale for Any Salad Bar is, of course, a variety of delicious salad dressings and flavorful dips, for nonfat tortilla chips, nonfat crackers, and vegetable sticks. (See **Dips, Spreads & Crudities**; and **Salad Dressings**.)

Notes: _____

Salad Dressings

General Guidelines for Making and Using Dressings

1. The easiest and fastest way to prepare salad dressings is by using a Vita-Mix machine. This eliminates the chopping and mincing steps. The ingredients can simply be thrown into the machine and it does the chopping, mincing, blending and emulsifying.

2. Dressings are best prepared at least 30 minutes prior to being served. The flavors need time to marinate. Overnight is even better.

3. Dressings will usually keep well for up to 1 week, if refrigerated and stored in a tightly covered bottle or container.

4. Shake the bottle well just before each use, as ingredients tend to separate when dressing is sitting for any length of time.

5. If you have just a little of two different dressings left, don't throw them out! Try mixing them for a new taste.

6. The following dressings are not limited to use on salads. Be adventurous and try various dressings on steamed vegetables, as well as baked, grilled or broiled fish, poultry and wild game meats.

Nonfat Tomato-Basil Dressing

1/2 cup low sodium tomato juice
Juice of 1/2 fresh lemon
1 tsp. pure maple syrup

2 medium cloves of garlic, minced
2 tsp. fresh basil, chopped
1 tsp. Spicy Mrs. Dash

Combine all of the ingredients and let sit, refrigerated, for at least 30 minutes, to marinate the flavors.

Notes: _____

Nonfat Herb Dressing

1/2 cup organic apple cider
1/4 cup white wine vinegar
3 medium cloves of garlic, minced
1 tsp. Spicy Mrs. Dash
2 scallions, finely chopped

1/2 tsp. dried basil
1/2 tsp. dried oregano
1/2 tsp. dried rosemary
1 tsp. Dijon mustard

Combine all of the ingredients and let sit, refrigerated, for about 30 minutes before use.

Lowfat Cheesy Herb Dressing

1 cup plain, nonfat yogurt
1 cup nonfat cottage cheese
4 tbsp. Parmesan or Romano cheese
2 scallions, chopped
2 medium cloves of garlic, minced

Juice of 1/2 fresh lemon
1 tbsp. pure maple syrup
1 tbsp. Dijon mustard
1 tsp. dried basil
1/8 - 1/4 tsp. hot pepper sauce

Either combine all of the ingredients in a blender, or use a Vita-Mix machine to save a lot of work and to provide a much smoother consistency. Chill thoroughly before use.

Nonfat Mustard Vinaigrette Dressing

1/4 cup apple cider vinegar
1/4 cup white wine vinegar
1 scallion, finely chopped
2 medium cloves of garlic, minced

1 tsp. black mustard seeds, ground
1/4 inch fresh ginger, grated
1 tsp. Dijon mustard
Mrs. Dash, to taste

Either combine all of the ingredients by hand, or save yourself some work and blend them together in a Vita-Mix machine.

Notes: _____

Nonfat Creamy Mustard-Yogurt Dressing

3/4 cup plain, nonfat yogurt
2 tbsp. dry mustard powder
Juice of 1/2 lemon

Mrs. Dash, to taste
Fresh ground pepper, to taste

In a blender, blend all of the ingredients together. Chill thoroughly before serving. Keeps about 2 - 3 days in refrigerator.

Vinaigrette Dressing

1/2 cup balsamic vinegar
1 tbsp. pure virgin olive oil
2 medium cloves of garlic, minced

2 tsp. Dijon mustard
1/4 - 1/2 tsp. fresh ground pepper

In a blender, blend all of the ingredients together. Chill thoroughly before serving.

French Dressing

1 tbsp. pure virgin olive oil
2 tbsp. fresh parsley, chopped
Juice of 3 fresh lemons
2 scallions, finely chopped
2 medium cloves of garlic, minced

1/4 tsp. dried rosemary
1/4 tsp. dried thyme
1/2 tsp. dried oregano
1/2 tsp. dried basil
1/8 tsp. paprika

Either combine all of the ingredients by hand, or use a Vita-Mix machine to save yourself some work. Chill thoroughly before serving.

Notes: _____

Cheesy Ginger Dressing

1 cup ricotta cheese
1/4 cup buttermilk
Juice of 1 fresh lemon
2 medium cloves of garlic (optional)

1/2 medium onion, chopped
1/2 inch fresh ginger root, grated
2 tbsp. pure maple syrup

In a blender, or Vita-Mix machine, blend all of the ingredients together until smooth and creamy. Chill thoroughly prior to serving.

Honey-Mustard Dressing

1/2 cup Nayonnaise
1/2 cup plain, nonfat yogurt
Juice of 1/2 fresh lemon

2 tbsp. Dijon mustard
1 tbsp. natural honey
1/4 tsp. fresh ground pepper

In a blender, blend all of the ingredients together. Chill for at least 30 minutes.

Variations: For **Honey-Lemon Dressing**, eliminate the mustard, and add the grated lemon rind from 1/2 lemon.

For **Lemon Dressing**, eliminate the honey or reduce to 1 tsp., use the juice of 1 whole lemon, and include the grated lemon rind from 1/2 lemon.

Green Goddess Buttermilk Dressing

1/2 cup buttermilk
1/2 cup Nayonnaise
Juice of 1/2 fresh lemon
2 tbsp. white wine vinegar

2 medium cloves of garlic, minced
1/4 cup fresh parsley, chopped
1/4 tsp. dried tarragon
1/4 tsp. fresh ground pepper

In a blender, blend all of the ingredients together until smooth. Chill thoroughly before use.

Notes: _____

Watercress Buttermilk Dressing

1/2 cup buttermilk
1/4 cup seasoned rice wine vinegar
2 scallions, chopped
2 medium cloves of garlic, chopped
1/2 cup watercress leaves, packed

1/4 tsp. fresh ground pepper
1/2 tsp. dried tarragon
1 tsp. pure maple syrup
1/2 tsp. Spicy Mrs. Dash
Rind of 1 lime (optional)

Either in a blender, or in a Vita-Mix machine (which will save you the work of chopping vegetables), blend all of the ingredients until smooth. Chill thoroughly before use.

Variation: For **Honey Dijon Watercress Dressing**, substitute the maple syrup with 1 tbsp. natural honey, eliminate the tarragon and the rind of a lime, and add 1 - 2 tbsp. of Dijon mustard.

Balsamic Garlic Dressing

2 tbsp. pure virgin olive oil
3/4 cup balsamic vinegar
5 medium cloves of garlic, minced

1/2 cup fresh parsley, chopped
1 tsp. Spicy Mrs. Dash

Either mix in a bottle or blend in a blender. Let sit in a covered glass bottle or jar, on a shelf that gets direct sunlight for at least half a day, to marinate the flavors.

Variation: For **Balsamic Dressing** (basic), reduce the garlic to 2 cloves and add 1/4 - 1/2 tsp. fresh ground pepper. Use the same procedure for preparation.

Spicy Dressing

1 tbsp. pure virgin olive oil
1/2 cup low sodium tomato juice
Juice of 1/2 fresh lemon
2 tbsp. organic cider vinegar
1/4 of large red onion, chopped
1/2 tsp. dry mustard powder

2 medium cloves of garlic, chopped
1/2 - 1 tsp. uncreamed horseradish
1/8 - 1/4 tsp. cayenne pepper
1/2 tsp. dried oregano
1 tbsp. pure maple syrup

In a blender, blend all of the ingredients together until smooth. Let sit for at least 1 hour before serving to enhance the blend of flavors.

Spicy Ginger Dressing

1 tbsp. pure virgin olive oil
1 tsp. sesame oil
Juice of 2 fresh limes
Rind of 1 lime, grated
3/4 - 1 inch fresh ginger root, grated

2 medium cloves garlic, minced
1/8 - 1/4 tsp. hot pepper sauce
1 tbsp. tamari sauce
1 tbsp. pure maple syrup

Either blend in a blender, or, for ease of preparation, use a Vita-Mix machine. Let sit for at least 1 hour before serving to enhance the blend of flavors.

Variation: For **Lemon-Ginger Dressing**, substitute the lime juice with the juice of 2 fresh lemons, and substitute the lime rind with the grated rind of 1 lemon.

Caesar Salad Dressing

This is best done in a Vita-Mix machine. Failing that, use a blender.

Because of the potential for salmonella poisoning from raw eggs, I have resorted to an egg substitute in this recipe. Since everything else in the recipe is fresh and natural, this is still a much more wholesome alternative than the many commercial varieties! And though there is some fat in this recipe, when divided into 6 servings, it is not enough to do any harm. And it's certainly a more healthy variety of oil than the hydrogenated oils used in the bottles of dressings found on the grocery store shelves! So go ahead and enjoy a treat!

2 tbsp. pure virgin olive oil
1/3 cup red wine vinegar
1/4 cup egg substitute
2 medium cloves of garlic, minced
1 tbsp. Dijon mustard

1/2 - 1 tsp. Spicy Mrs. Dash
1/4 - 1/2 tsp. fresh ground pepper
3 tbsp. Parmesan or Romano cheese
1/4 - 1/2 tsp. hot pepper sauce
2 tsp. anchovy paste

In a Vita-Mix machine, or blender, blend all of the ingredients together until very smooth. Cover and chill thoroughly before serving.

Variation: For **Nonfat Caesar Dressing**, eliminate the oil and anchovy paste, and use nonfat Parmesan cheese by Alpine Lace.

Tofu Curry Dressing

8 ounces soft tofu
1 tsp. sesame oil
Juice of 1 fresh lemon
1 tbsp. natural honey
2 medium cloves of garlic, minced

1 tsp. curry powder
1/2 inch fresh ginger root, grated
1 tsp. Spicy Mrs. Dash
1/8 - 1/4 tsp. hot pepper sauce (optional)

Either in a blender or a Vita-Mix machine, blend all of the ingredients together until very smooth. Chill thoroughly prior to serving.

Mock Sour Cream Dressing

8 ounces soft tofu
2 tbsp. pure virgin olive oil
Juice of 1/2 fresh lemon

2 tsp. pure maple syrup
1 tsp. Mrs. Dash

In a blender, blend all of the ingredients together until smooth. Use in recipes which call for sour cream, or use as is, as a topping or dressing.

Salsa-Yogurt Dressing

1/2 cup plain, nonfat yogurt
1/2 cup fresh, medium salsa
2 medium cloves of garlic, chopped

Juice of 1 fresh lime
3 scallions, finely chopped

Mix all of the ingredients together. Chill thoroughly prior to use.

Note: Many grocery stores and health food stores carry fresh salsa, made daily, in their deli sections. These are the only ones I buy! Avoid those almost dead brands which sit on the shelves forever without needing refrigeration! Remember, fresh is best!

Notes: _____

Seasoned Yogurt and Tofu Topping

1 cup (8 ounces) soft tofu	1 tbsp. pure maple syrup
1/2 cup plain, nonfat yogurt	1 tbsp. Bragg's Liquid Aminos
2 medium cloves of garlic, minced	1/8 to 1/4 tsp. hot pepper sauce
Juice of 1 fresh lemon	1/4 cup fresh parsley, chopped

In a blender or a Vita-Mix machine, blend all of the ingredients until smooth. Chill thoroughly prior to use.

Variation: For **Tuna and Seasoned Yogurt**, substitute the tofu with 6 ounces of water-packed canned tuna, well drained and rinsed. And eliminate the maple syrup. *This a high protein, high omega-3, EPA topping for baked potatoes, as well as a great dip or dressing for other vegetables.*

Miso Dressing

1 cup of soft tofu	2 medium cloves of garlic, minced
2 tbsp. red miso paste	1 tbsp. pure maple syrup
1 tbsp. pure olive oil	1/2 tsp. paprika
Juice of 1 fresh lemon	

In a blender, blend all of the ingredients until smooth. Chill prior to serving.

Note: For **Miso Spread**, substitute the soft tofu with very firm tofu, and the maple syrup with sucanat.

Tahini and Buttermilk Dressing

1/2 cup buttermilk	1 tsp. Spicy Mrs. Dash
1/4 cup sesame tahini	1/2 tsp. fresh ground pepper
2 medium cloves of garlic, minced	1/4 tsp. dry mustard powder
Juice of 1/2 fresh lemon	

In a blender, blend all of the ingredients together thoroughly. Chill prior to serving.

High Omega-3 GLA Dressing

1 tbsp. cold pressed flaxseed oil
1 tsp. sesame oil
Juice of 2 fresh lemons
Rind of 1 lemon, grated
1/8 tsp. hot pepper sauce

2 medium cloves of garlic, minced
1/2 inch fresh ginger root, grated
1 tbsp. Bragg's Liquid Aminos
1 tsp. Mrs. Dash

In a blender, blend all of the ingredients together thoroughly. Let flavors marinate prior to serving.

Note: **Flaxseed Oil** *can be substituted for any of the oils used in the various dressing recipes.* However, be aware of the fact that it does have a particular flavor that is not as readily accepted as that of other oils. The good news is that with continued use, a taste for this oil can be acquired. After a few years of regular use and a lot of experimentation with recipes, I actually enjoy the flavor now. Of course the fact that it is so beneficial to my body's health makes it all the more enjoyable to me!

Mustard Yogurt Dressing

1/2 cup plain, nonfat yogurt
1/4 cup Nayonnaise

1/2 small onion, finely chopped
1½ - 2 tbsp. Dijon mustard

Mix the ingredients together thoroughly. Cover and refrigerate.

Variation: For **Dill Yogurt Dressing**, substitute the Dijon mustard with 1 tsp. dried dill weed. Cover and refrigerate.

Notes: _____

Marinades

General Guidelines For Using Marinades

1. Marinades can be used for enhancing the flavor of firm to very firm tofu, fish, poultry and vegetables.

2   Generally the longer the marinating time, the better the flavor of the finished product.

3. Marinate tofu and fish for a minimum of 2 - 4 hours, preferably overnight.

4. Marinate chicken and turkey, and most game meats for a minimum of 4 - 6 hours, preferably overnight.

5   Marinate most vegetables for about 1 - 4 hours before eating as they are, or cooking them. Vegetables with a lower water content are the best for marinating.

6. Vegetable sticks can be placed in a ziplock baggie or a tightly sealed container, with some marinade, and carried to the office or on a hiking trip, for a flavorful addition to a meal or as a snack.

7. Most marinades keep well, in the refrigerator, for up to 1 week, in a tightly sealed jar or container.

8. Marinades with a yogurt or buttermilk base, are best used within 2 - 3 days.

Teriyaki Marinade

1 tbsp. minced fresh ginger
3 medium cloves of garlic, minced
1 tbsp. pure maple syrup
3 scallions, finely chopped
1/2 cup Bragg's Liquid Aminos

Juice of 1 large fresh lemon
1 tbsp. sesame oil
1/4 - 1/2 tsp. hot pepper sauce
1/4 cup of white wine (optional)
1/4 cup water

Combine all ingredients and keep in tightly sealed jar in refrigerator.

Notes: _____

Herb Marinade

1 tbsp. pure virgin olive oil
1/4 cup balsamic vinegar
Juice of 1 large fresh lemon
1 tsp. Spicy Mrs. Dash
3 medium cloves of garlic, chopped
1/2 medium onion, finely chopped

1/4 - 1/2 tsp. hot pepper sauce
1/4 cup fresh parsley, chopped
1 tsp. dried rosemary
1 tsp. dried dill
1 tsp. dried tarragon
2 tbsp. hot water

1.   Soak the dried herbs in hot water while preparing the rest of the marinade.
2.   Combine the remaining ingredients.
3.   Add the dried herbs and their soaking water to the combined ingredients.
4.   Store in a tightly sealed jar in the refrigerator.

French-Style Marinade

3 medium cloves of garlic, minced
3 scallions, finely chopped
1 tbsp. pure virgin olive oil
1/2 cup red wine vinegar
1 tsp. Spicy Mrs. Dash
1/4 cup water

2 tsp. dried oregano
1 tbsp. Dijon mustard
1 tbsp. pure maple syrup
1/8 to 1/4 tsp. ground red pepper
1/8 - 1/4 tsp. sherry extract

Combine all of the ingredients and store in a tightly sealed jar in refrigerator.

Sweet and Sour Marinade

1/2 cup pineapple juice
1/2 cup organic cider vinegar
2 medium cloves of garlic, sliced
3 scallions, finely chopped
2 tbsp. pure maple syrup

Rind of 1 lemon, grated
1/2 cup fresh parsley, chopped
1/2 tsp. dry mustard powder
1/8 - 1/4 tsp. hot pepper sauce

Combine all of the ingredients and store in a tightly sealed jar in refrigerator.

Minty Yogurt Marinade

3/4 cup plain, nonfat yogurt
Juice of 1 fresh lime
Rind of 1 lime, grated
3 medium cloves of garlic, minced
3 scallions, finely chopped

1/4 cup fresh parsley, chopped
1/8 - 1/4 tsp. hot pepper sauce
1/2 tsp. caraway seeds
1 tsp. mint, finely chopped

Combine all of the ingredients and store in a tightly sealed jar in refrigerator. Use within 2 - 3 days.

Garlic-Tomato Marinade

1/2 cup low sodium tomato juice
Juice of 1 large fresh lemon
1/4 cup water
4 medium cloves of garlic, chopped
1/2 medium onion, finely chopped

1/4 - 1/2 tsp. dry mustard powder
1/4 cup fresh cilantro, chopped
1/8 - 1/4 tsp. ground red pepper
1 tbsp. pure virgin olive oil (optional)

Combine all of the ingredients and store in a tightly sealed jar in refrigerator.

The Drunken Limey Marinade

Juice of 2 fresh limes
Rind of 1 lime, grated
1/2 cup dry white wine
3 medium cloves of garlic, minced
1 tbsp. pure maple syrup

1/2 medium onion, finely chopped
1/2 inch fresh ginger root, grated
1/4 tsp. nutmeg
1/4 - 1/2 tsp. hot pepper sauce

Combine all of the ingredients and store in a tightly sealed jar in refrigerator.

Notes:

Main Entrees

Turkey Loaf

1 lb. ground turkey breast
1 medium onion, chopped
1/2 medium green pepper, chopped
1/2 medium red pepper, chopped
2 medium cloves of garlic, minced
1 free-range egg

3/4 cup old fashioned oatmeal
1/4 cup wheat germ
1 cup Pomi tomatoes, crushed*
1 tbsp. Mrs. Dash or Spicy Mrs. Dash
1 tsp. dried oregano
1/4 tsp. fresh ground pepper

1.   Thoroughly combine all of the ingredients.
2.   Form into a loaf shape, and then place in a loaf pan or dish.
3.   Bake at 350º for 40 - 45 minutes. Let stand for 5 minutes before serving.
4.   Serve with **Mustard Yogurt Dressing.**

* Pomi tomatoes come in a carton containing 26 ounces of tomatoes. They are vacuum packed fresh, with no salt, no preservatives, no water added, and no artificial flavoring. *This is the only way I will buy tomatoes, other than fresh!*
Pomi tomatoes are available in most grocery stores, health food stores and drugmarts, such as Savon or Thrifty's. (See **References and Resources.**)

Makes 4 - 6 servings

Vegetarian Chili

1 medium onion, chopped
2 large carrots, sliced
1 stalk celery, chopped
4 medium cloves of garlic, minced
1 medium green pepper, chopped
1 medium red pepper, chopped
2 fresh jalapenos, chopped#
1 cup water or vegetable stock*

2 tbsp. chili powder#
1 carton (26 ounces) Pomi tomatoes
1 tsp. cumin
2 tsp. Spicy Mrs. Dash
1/2 tsp. fresh ground pepper
1 can (16 ounces) pinto beans, drained
2 tbsp. fresh cilantro, finely chopped

1.   In a Dutch oven, combine all of the ingredients, except cilantro.
2.   Bring the chili to a simmer. Cover and simmer for 20 - 30 minutes, or until vegetables are tender, but not mushy.
3.   Stir in the cilantro and serve.

* For a healthy natural **Vegetable Stock**, to use in cooking, I collect all of the leftover liquid from steaming vegetables. I store it in an airtight glass jar in the refrigerator and use this instead of commercial canned stocks, which are generally loaded with sodium and often contain less than healthy fat sources. At the end of 1 week, whatever stock is still remaining, I throw out. After the jar is thoroughly washed, I begin collecting stock again.
Note: *There is rarely any stock left at the end of each week.*

If you are not used to hot food, or rarely eat spicy foods, you may want to reduce the chili powder to 1 tbsp. the first time you make this chili. You can always add more the next time you make it. *But you can't eliminate the heat after it has already been added!*
Note: *Experiment with the jalapeno peppers as well*. Start with only 1 pepper and then add more as you tolerate it. Make the recipe *work for you* and your tastebuds!

Makes 4 servings

Notes: _____

Vegetable-Tofu Medley

1 medium onion, sliced	1 cup fresh broccoli, chopped
2 medium cloves of garlic, minced	1/2 lb. extra firm tofu, diced
1 medium green pepper, sliced	1/2 inch fresh ginger, grated
1 medium red pepper, sliced	1 - 2 tbsp. water or vegetable stock
1 cup fresh mushrooms, sliced	1 tbsp. low sodium soy sauce
1 fresh carrot, sliced	1 tsp. sesame oil

1. To a hot wok or large skillet, add the sesame oil, soy sauce, stock and ginger.

2. When mixture is steaming, add all of vegetables. Saute briefly, just to heat vegetables, but not to cook them

3. Add tofu and toss quickly over the heat.

4. Serve over brown rice or wholegrain noodles. Great topped with a sprinkling of fresh ground pepper.

Makes 4 servings.

Notes:

Wholegrain Pasta / High Protein Marinara Sauce

#1 - The Quickie Version

1 - 26 ounce bottle natural, lowfat, garlic and mushroom marinara sauce
8 - 10 ounces soft tofu

1. In a saucepan, heat the sauce until just beginning to bubble.
2. Using a potato masher, mash the tofu into the marinara sauce.
3. Remove saucepan from heat just as the mixture begins to form bubbles again. *Do not cook the tofu!*
4. Serve over wholegrain or vegetable pasta. Also good served over brown rice.

#2 - From Scratch (Almost!)

1/4 cup water
1 tsp. vegetable seasoning powder
2 medium cloves of garlic, minced
1 medium onion, chopped
1/4 cup fresh parsley, chopped

1 carton (26 ounces) Pomi tomatoes
1 tsp. dried oregano
1/3 cup fresh basil, chopped
1/4 tsp. chili pepper flakes
8 - 10 ounces soft tofu
2 tbsp. Parmesan cheese, optional

1. Put all ingredients, except the tofu and Parmesan cheese, into a saucepan.
2. Simmer gently for 25 - 30 minutes.
3. Using a potato masher, mash the tofu into the marinara sauce.
4. Remove saucepan from heat just as mixture begins to form bubbles again. *Do not cook the tofu!*
5. Stir Parmesan into sauce until well combined. Serve over pasta or rice.

Variation: For **Tofu-Mushroom Marinara Sauce,** prepare as for Marinara **#2 - From Scratch,** adding 1 cup of sliced fresh mushrooms in the first step, and following as listed, steps #2 through #5.

Note: **If you have a Vita-Mix machine,** this recipe is a cinch! *Don't waste any time chopping or mincing!* Just throw all of the ingredients, except the tofu and Parmesan, into the Vita-Mix. Blend on high speed for about 1 minute. The action of the machine heats the food while it blends it. Then add the tofu and Parmesan and blend very briefly for about 5 - 10 seconds. Serve immediately.

Bean Burritos with Salsa and Yogurt

One of the quickest meals I know!

1. Spoon some black beans (come in 16 ounce cans), slightly off center onto a corn or wholewheat tortilla.

2. Sprinkle some grated nonfat cheese over the beans, and a spoonful each of chunky salsa, and of plain, nonfat yogurt.

3. Fold the short sides of the tortilla over the filling. Then fold over the long sides, placing the seam side down on the plate.

4. They taste best when served warm. Serve with a salad of greens and tomatoes.

Baked Chicken Breast / Baked Turkey Breast

3 - 4 skinless, boneless chicken
  or turkey breasts
1/4 tsp. black pepper
1 cup raw oatmeal, slightly ground
1 tsp. minced garlic

1 tsp. Mrs. Dash
1/4 - 1/2 tsp. Worcestershire sauce
1 egg white
1/4 tsp. hot pepper sauce

1. Whip together all of ingredients but chicken and oatmeal.
2. Roll chicken breast in egg white mixture and then coat with oatmeal.
3. Bake chicken breasts at 400° for 20-25 minutes; bake longer for turkey breasts.
4. Serve with brown rice, and a fresh green salad with nonfat, or low fat, dressing.
5. To toast the oatmeal, broil the chicken briefly, after actual baking is completed. It browns the coating nicely.

Note: If the oatmeal is initially ground slightly in a coffee mill, the consistency will be similar to bread crumbs and will therefore, more easily, become crispy during the baking period, eliminating the need to use the broiler.

Makes 3 - 4 servings.

Pasta and Vegetable Medley

A very simple dish for the end of a crazy work day, or for a community potluck dinner!

1 lb. wholegrain or vegetable pasta, elbows or bow ties	1/4 cup Nayonnaise
1 lb. frozen mixed vegetables, Mediterranean blend	1/2 cup plain, nonfat yogurt
4 scallions, finely chopped	2 tbsp. Dijon mustard
2 large cloves of garlic, minced	1/2 tsp. fresh ground pepper
1/2 cup pitted black olives, chopped	1 tsp. dried basil
1 can (16 ounces) chickpeas, drained	1/4 cup fresh parsley, chopped
	Hot pepper sauce, to taste

1. Cook pasta according to directions on package. Drain.
2. Cook frozen vegetables according to directions on package. Drain.
3. In a separate bowl, combine all of seasoning ingredients in the second column.
4. Combine pasta, vegetables, scallions, garlic, olives, chickpeas and seasoning mixture. Toss until thoroughly mixed.
5. Cover and refrigerate for at least 60 minutes prior to serving, to blend flavors.

Variations: 1. To increase protein, add marinated tofu chunks, tuna, salmon, or chunks of chicken breast or leftover cooked fish.

2. To serve hot, put mixture into a lightly sprayed pyrex casserole dish and bake at 350° for about 20 minutes.

Makes 6 servings.

Notes:

Chicken Fajitas - Quick and Healthy!

Less cooking!   More Crunch!   Higher nutrition!

1½ lb. cooked skinless chicken breast
1 tbsp. pure virgin olive oil
3 medium cloves of garlic, minced
1 large red onion, thinly sliced
1 large green pepper, in thin strips
1 large red pepper, in thin strips

1/4 tsp. cayenne pepper
1/2 - 1 cup fresh salsa
1/2 medium avocado, thinly sliced
1/2 - 1 cup nonfat, plain yogurt
Cheddar cheese, nonfat, shredded
8 whole wheat tortillas, heated

1. Cut chicken into thin strips.
2. Place tortillas in covered pyrex dish in preheated 250° oven for about 10 minutes.
3. Heat oil in large skillet. Add garlic, onions, peppers, cayenne pepper and chicken.
4. Saute over medium heat for about 5 minutes.
5. To assemble fajitas spoon the vegetable and chicken mixture down center of the tortilla. Top with a spoonful of salsa, a slice of avocado, a spoonful of yogurt, and a sprinkling of shredded cheese. Encase filling by folding like an envelope, leaving one end open.
6. Serve with Mexican Brown Rice.

Makes 8 servings.

Sweet Potato and Vegetable Casserole

3 medium sweet potatoes, unpeeled
    cut into slices
1 medium onion, chopped
3 medium carrots, sliced
2 small zucchini, in chunks
2 stalks celery, chopped
1 carton (26 ounces) Pomi tomatoes
1 cup fresh green beans

1 can (16 ounces) red kidney beans
2 tbsp. pure maple syrup
1 tsp. dried oregano
1 tsp. dried basil
1/2 tsp. dried thyme
1/8 - 1/4 tsp. hot pepper sauce
Plain, nonfat yogurt, optional
Parmesan or Romano cheese, optional

1. In a large bowl, toss all ingredients to mix thoroughly.
2. Spoon into a pyrex casserole dish, sprayed with olive oil-based cooking spray.
3. Bake at 350° for about 30 minutes.
4. Can serve topped with plain, nonfat yogurt and a sprinkling of Parmesan cheese.

Makes 4 servings.

Light Whole Wheat Macaroni and Cheese

2 cups uncooked whole wheat
    elbow macaroni
2 medium cloves of garlic, minced
1 tsp. dry mustard
1 tsp. dried basil
1/2 tsp. paprika

1 - 1½ tbsp. Molly McButter
1/2 cup nonfat, plain yogurt
8 ounces Cheddar cheese, nonfat,
    shredded
3 tbsp. rolled oats, ground
2 tbsp. fresh parsley, chopped

1. Cook macaroni to desired firmness as directed on the package. Drain.
2. Add garlic, seasonings, Molly McButter, yogurt and cheese. Mix well.
3. Spoon into ungreased pyrex casserole dish. Top with oats, ground in coffee mill.
4. Bake at 350° for 25 minutes. Sprinkle with chopped parsley.

Variations: Tuna, salmon, crabmeat, shrimp, or other fish or shellfish, chopped skinless chicken or turkey breast, black beans or other legumes, cooked broccoli, snowpeas or green beans, or any assortment of these ingredients can be added to the casserole prior to baking in the oven.

Makes 4 - 6 servings.

Notes:

Fresh Baked Trout with Lemon

1½ lb. boneless trout fillets
1/2 cup low sodium soy sauce
1/2 cup white wine

2 tbsp. pure maple syrup
1 - 1½ inches fresh ginger, grated
1 medium onion, thinly sliced

1. Mix all ingredients except the trout together and pour into pyrex baking dish.
2. Place trout in the mixture, cover and refrigerate.
3. Let marinate 30 minutes on each side before cooking.
4. Bake at 400º for 12 - 15 minutes, or until fish flakes easily when tested with a fork.
5. Pour marinade and baking juices over each serving. Serve with fresh lemon wedges and fresh ground black pepper..

Note: The alcohol content in the wine is cooked off during the baking of the fish.

Makes 4 servings.

Mexican Brown Rice

2 medium onions, chopped
1 large green pepper, chopped
2 large cloves of garlic, minced
1/2 carton (13 ounces) Pomi tomatoes

3 cups boiling water
2 tbsp. vegetable seasoning powder
2 cups uncooked brown rice
2 tbsp. fresh parsley, chopped

1. Put all ingredients into a heavy saucepan and bring to a boil.
2. Cover, reduce heat and simmer on low heat for about 40 - 45 minutes, or until all of the liquid is absorbed.

Makes 4 - 6 servings.

Notes:

Turkey Chili

1 lb. ground turkey breast	1 tsp. dried oregano
1 carton (26 ounces) Pomi tomatoes	1/2 tsp. dried basil
2 medium unpeeled potatoes, diced	1 tsp. Spicy Mrs. Dash
1 large onion, chopped	1 - 2 tbsp. chili powder
3 large cloves of garlic, minced	1/4 tsp. fresh ground pepper
1/2 large green pepper, chopped	2 cans (16 ounces each) red kidney
1 or 2 fresh jalapenos, chopped	beans, drained and rinsed

1. Put all of the ingredients except kidney beans into a Dutch oven. Mix thoroughly.
2. Bring to a boil, then cover, reduce heat and simmer for about 20 minutes.
3. Add kidney beans and simmer for another 10 minutes.
4. Can be topped with plain, nonfat yogurt and served in a variety of ways:

    a. with wholegrain bread or toast
    b. over brown rice, or other cooked grains
    c. as a dip for baked tortilla chips or nonfat wholegrain crackers
    d. as a topping on a tostada salad
    e. in a taco shell and topped with leafy greens, salsa and yogurt
    f. as a filling for a burrito

Makes 8 - 10 servings.

Steamed Bulgur with Nonfat Yogurt

1 cup raw bulgur	1 cup plain, nonfat yogurt
1 3/4 cups boiling water	
or vegetable broth	

1. Place bulgur in a large bowl. Pour boiling liquid over bulgur.
2. Cover and let sit until grain has absorbed all of liquid, about 20 - 25 minutes.
3. Thoroughly blend yogurt throughout the bulgur, and serve.

Note: Any grain lends itself to preparation with vegetable broth and the addition of yogurt.

Makes 4 servings.

Curried Vegetables and Imitation Crabmeat

1 cup water, boiling
1 tbsp. vegetable seasoning powder
1 medium onion, chopped
2 medium cloves of garlic, minced
4 medium potatoes, unpeeled, chopped
1/2 lb. fresh cauliflower, chopped
2 medium carrots, chopped

1 cup fresh or frozen green peas
2 tbsp. curry powder
1 tsp. dried basil
1 tsp. sucanat
1/2 cup nonalcoholic, or dry, wine
1/2 cup plain, nonfat yogurt
1 lb. imitation crabmeat, flaked

1. Add the vegetable seasoning powder, eg. brands by Gayelord Hauser or Bernard Jensen, to the boiling water. Mix thoroughly.
2. Place all but 2 tbsp. of the broth into a Dutch oven. Add all of the vegetables to the broth.
3. Blend curry powder well with 2 tbsp. broth. Mix with basil, sucanat, and wine.
4. Add the curry mixture to the vegetables and broth in the Dutch oven.
5. Bring to a boil. Cover, reduce heat and simmer about 20 minutes or until vegetables are tender, but not soft.
6. Stir the yogurt and flaked crabmeat throughout the vegetable mixture. Heat through, but do not bring to a boil.
7. Serve over steamed bulgur, plain, or mixed with yogurt. Also great with brown rice.

Variations:
1. Fresh steamed crabmeat can be used instead of imitation crabmeat.

2. Cooked, diced chicken, or turkey, breast can be substituted for the crabmeat.

3. A mixture of steamed shrimps, lobster and crabmeat can be substituted.

4. Any whitefish can be substituted for the crabmeat. Either steam the fish and cut into 1" or 2" pieces, prior to adding it to the curried vegetables. Or add raw fillets, cut into 1" or 2" pieces, 3 - 4 minutes prior to end of cooking time.

Makes 6 - 8 servings.

Notes: _____

Vegetable and Bean Chili

1 medium onion, chopped
4 medium cloves of garlic, minced
1 carton (26 ounces) Pomi tomatoes
1 medium green pepper, chopped
1 medium red pepper, chopped
2 large carrots, sliced
1/2 lb. fresh broccoli, chopped

2 fresh jalapenos, chopped
2 tbsp. chili powder
1 tsp. cumin
1 - 2 tsp. Mrs. Dash
1/2 tsp. fresh ground pepper
1 can (16 ounces) red kidney beans, drained
1/4 cup fresh cilantro, chopped

1. In a Dutch oven, put all ingredients except the cilantro.
2. Bring the chili to a simmer. Continue to simmer for 20 - 30 minutes.
3. Stir in the cilantro and serve.
4. Delicious served with fresh wholegrain cornbread. Also great over brown rice, or other grains.

Makes 4 servings.

Fettucini Alfredo for Health

Whole wheat or vegetable pasta noodles
1/2 - 1 tsp. Spicy Mrs. Dash
1 - 2 tsp. garlic-flavored Molly McButter

2 - 4 tbsp. Parmesan cheese
1/4 - 1/2 cup plain nonfat yogurt
Fresh ground pepper
Juice of 1/2 lemon, squeezed

1. Cook enough pasta for 2 - 4 servings, according to directions on package.
2. Drain pasta, and add Molly McButter, Parmesan cheese, Mrs. Dash, yogurt and lemon juice.
3. Toss pasta.
4. Serve with fresh ground pepper sprinkled on top, to taste. Excellent with a fresh green salad and steamed vegetables.

Makes 2 - 4 servings.

Notes:

Seasoned Baked Potato Wedges

These can be done from scratch, or using previously baked potatoes!

#1 - The Quickie Version

Olive oil-based cooking spray
6 medium baked potatoes, unpeeled*
All natural flavor spray,
    eg. Mesquite Mist

1/4 cup fresh thyme, rosemary, dill,
    basil or parsley, chopped
Fresh ground black pepper, to taste

1. Cut the previously baked potatoes into 1/2" wedges.
2. Spray a baking sheet with nonstick cooking spray.
3. Arrange the potato wedges on the baking sheet, with space between the wedges.
4. Spray the surface of the wedges lightly with an all natural flavor spray of your choice.
5. Sprinkle the thyme, or other herbs, and black pepper over all of the potato pieces.
6. Grill briefly under the broiler, for about 4 - 5 minutes, or until wedges turn golden brown and slightly crispy on the outside, and are hot in the center.

*When I bake potatoes for a meal, I bake 10 - 20 potatoes at the same time. Saves energy! Fuel energy, as well as personal energy! Whatever is not eaten at the meal is covered and stored in the refrigerator for "near"-future meals. Some of the leftover potatoes may be used to make these potato wedges, others may be used to make a potato salad to carry to a potluck dinner, and others may simply be carried in the car for a nutritious emergency snack!

#2 - The Scratch Version

Olive oil-based cooking spray
6 medium potatoes, scrubbed, unpeeled
All natural flavor spray, of choice

1/4 cup fresh thyme, rosemary, dill,
    basil or parsley, chopped
Paprika

1. Preheat oven to 450°.
2. Cut potatoes into 1/2" wedges and arrange on lightly sprayed baking sheet.
3. Spray the surface of the wedges lightly with an all natural flavor spray of your choice.
4. Sprinkle the thyme, or other herbs, and paprika over all of the potato pieces.
5. Bake for 30 - 40 minutes, until the wedges are golden brown and crispy on the outside, and tender on the inside. Loosen the wedges from the pan once or twice during the baking period with a spatula.

Each recipe makes 4 - 6 servings.

Spicy Beans and Vegetable Stew

1 medium onion, chopped	1 inch fresh ginger, grated
4 medium cloves of garlic, minced	1 tsp. paprika
1 cup vegetable stock or water	1 tsp. dried oregano
1 carton (26 ounces) Pomi tomatoes	1 tsp. dried thyme
1/2 lb. fresh cauliflower, chopped	1 tsp. ground cumin
1/2 lb. fresh broccoli, chopped	1/2 tsp. fresh ground pepper
2 stalks celery, chopped	1/4 tsp. cayenne pepper
1 large green pepper, chopped	2 tbsp. low sodium soy sauce
3 medium zucchini, sliced	1 can (16 ounces) chickpeas, drained
1 cup fresh mushrooms, halved	1 can (16 ounces) black beans, drained

1. Put all ingredients, except zucchini, soy sauce and beans, into a Dutch oven. Bring to a boil.
2. Cover, reduce heat and simmer for 15 - 20 minutes.
3. Add zucchini, drained chickpeas and black beans to the stew.
4. Cover, and simmer, until zucchini is tender, but not soft. About 10 minutes.
5. Stir soy sauce into finished stew. Serve over steamed millet, or brown rice.

Variation: For **Spicy Potatoes, Broccoli and Blackeyed Peas**, eliminate the tomatoes, cauliflower, celery and zucchini. Instead use 5 medium potatoes, unpeeled and chopped, and increase the broccoli to 1 lb. Substitute the chickpeas and black beans with 2 cans (16 ounces each) blackeyed peas, drained.

Note: This stew tastes even better the next day, after the flavors have had more time to blend together.

Makes 6 - 8 servings.

Notes:

Salmon Burger on Whole Wheat Kaiser Roll

2 cans (7.5 ounces each) salmon, drained and rinsed
1/2 cup rolled oats, coarsely ground
1/2 large onion, chopped
1 egg, free range

1/4 cup plain, nonfat yogurt
1½ tsp. dried dill weed
1 tsp. dry mustard
1/2 tsp. fresh ground pepper
Olive oil-based cooking spray

1. In a medium bowl, combine all ingredients. Mix well.
2. Shape mixture into 6 patties.
3. Spray large nonstick skillet with nonfat cooking spray.
4. Cook patties over medium heat for 6 - 8 minutes. Turn once during cooking.
5. Serve on whole wheat kaiser rolls, topped with any or all of the following:

red onion slices	tomato slices	lettuce
zucchini slices	cucumber slices	salsa
Dijon mustard	Nayonnaise	alfalfa sprouts
yogurt mustard dressing	red and green peppers	jalapenos

Notes:

Tofu-Vegetable Frittata

Olive oil-based cooking spray
1 large onion, thinly sliced
2 medium cloves of garlic, minced
1 large green pepper, thinly sliced
1 medium zucchini, sliced
1 large tomato, chopped
2 baked potatoes, unpeeled, chopped

8 ounces soft tofu, mashed
2 eggs, free range
1/4 tsp. turmeric
1 - 2 tsp. Mrs. Dash
1 tsp. dried basil
1/8 - 1/4 tsp. hot pepper sauce
4 ounces cheddar cheese, nonfat, shredded

1. Spray large nonstick oven-proof skillet with nonfat cooking spray.
2. Add all of ingredients in the first column and saute at medium heat for 3 - 4 minutes.
3. Mix together thoroughly all of ingredients in the second column. Pour over vegetable mixture.
4. Place skillet in preheated 350° oven. Bake 20 - 25 minutes, or until knife inserted in the center comes out clean.
5. Cut into pie-shaped wedges to serve.

Makes 4 - 6 servings.

Curried Chickpeas and Onions

1 cup water
1 tbsp. pure virgin olive oil
2 medium onions, sliced
2 medium cloves of garlic, minced
1 medium tomato, chopped
1/2 inch fresh ginger, grated
1½ tsp. coriander
1 tsp. cumin

1 bay leaf
1/2 tsp. turmeric
1 tsp. mustard seeds
1/4 tsp. cayenne pepper
1/2 tsp. Real Salt
3 medium potatoes, chopped
2 cans (16 ounces each) chickpeas, drained
Juice of 1 fresh lemon

1. Heat oil in medium-sized saucepan. Add all of ingredients except water, potatoes, chickpeas and lemon juice.
2. Saute mixture until mustard seeds begin to pop, about 3 - 5 minutes.
3. Add water, potatoes and chickpeas. Bring to a boil.
4. Cover, reduce heat, and simmer for about 20 minutes.
5. Remove from heat. Add lemon juice. Cover. Let sit for 10 minutes prior to serving.
6. Serve over steamed bulgur or brown rice.

Makes 4 servings.

Wholegrain Pasta Primavera

Olive oil-based cooking spray
1 medium red onion, coarsely chopped
3 medium cloves of garlic, minced
2 medium zucchini, sliced
1 large green pepper, sliced
1 large red pepper, sliced
1 cup fresh snowpeas
4 medium tomatoes, chopped
1/4 cup water

2 tsp. dried basil
1 tsp. dried oregano
1/2 tsp. dried thyme
1/4 cup nonalcoholic or regular
    white wine
1/2 tsp. Real Salt, optional
1/4 tsp. crushed red pepper flakes
6 - 8 ounces wholegrain linguine
Parmesan or Romano cheese

1. Prepare pasta according to directions on package.
2. Spray medium-sized saucepan with nonfat cooking spray.
3. Over medium-high heat, briefly saute onions and garlic, about 3 - 4 minutes.
4. Add rest of ingredients, except linguine and cheese. Simmer uncovered for 5 - 8 minutes. Vegetables should remain very crisp.
5. Serve sauce over cooked linguine. Lightly sprinkle cheese over sauce.

Makes 6 servings.

Seasoned Buckwheat Groats (also called Kasha)

1 cup whole buckwheat groats (kasha)
1 small onion, diced
2 medium cloves of garlic, minced

2 cups boiling water
2 tbsp. vegetable seasoning powder
1/4 cup sun-dried tomatoes, chopped

1. In a sieve, rinse kasha well under cool running water. Drain.
2. Put all ingredients into a medium-sized saucepan. Bring back to a boil.
3. Cover, reduce heat, and simmer until kasha is soft, about 12 - 15 minutes.
4. Remove from heat and let sit covered, and untouched, for 5 minutes.
5. Serve with **Baked Red Snapper**, or as is, topped with a serving of beans.

Makes 4 servings.

Notes: _____

Baked Red Snapper with Gingery Pineapple Sauce

Olive oil-based cooking spray
1½ lb. skinless Red Snapper fillets
1 tsp. sesame oil
1 medium onion, diced
2 medium cloves of garlic

1 cup fresh pineapple
1 - 2 tsp. pure maple syrup
3/4 inch fresh ginger, grated
1/8 - 1/4 tsp. hot pepper sauce
1 tbsp. tamari sauce

1.   Place the fillets in a shallow baking dish that has been sprayed.
2.   Blend the rest of the ingredients together in a blender or Vita- mix machine. The Vita-Mix saves you the task of chopping and mincing!
3.   Pour the sauce over the fillets. Cover and refrigerate for 30 - 60 minutes.
4.   Bake fish, in marinade, in preheated oven at 450° for 8 - 10 minutes, or just until fish flakes easily.
5.   Pour some of sauce from the baking dish, over each serving.

Makes 4 - 6 servings.

Salmon Loaf with Mustard Sauce

1 can (15 ounces) water-packed
        salmon, drained and rinsed
1 egg, free range
1/2 cup plain, nonfat yogurt
1 cup rolled oats, coarsely ground
1/2 large onion, diced

1 medium tomato, chopped
1½ tsp. curry powder
1 tsp. tarragon
1/4 cup fresh parsley, chopped
1 tsp. Mrs. Dash
1/4 tsp. fresh ground pepper
Olive oil-based cooking spray

1.   Mix all ingredients together well, except spray.
2.   Spray a nonstick loaf pan with nonfat cooking spray, and fill with salmon mixture.
3.   Bake in preheated 400° over for 20 - 25 minutes. Let sit for 10 minutes.
4.   Serve with a mustard dressing of your choice. See **Dressings** section.

Makes 4 - 6 servings.

Notes: _____

Dips, Spreads, Crudities

Evening with Friends

Raw Vegetable Platter
Green peppers, tomatoes, mushrooms, broccoli, cauliflower, zucchini, carrots, celery, etc.

Baked Tortilla Chips

DIP 1:   **Chunky Blend**

1/2 cup medium salsa
1/2 cup plain, nonfat yoghurt
1/2 cup nonfat cottage cheese
1 tsp. minced garlic

Put all ingredients together in a bowl. Mix well and let marinate in refrigerator for at least 2 hours.

DIP 2:   **Smooth Blend**

Above ingredients (Dip #1) + extra 1/4 cup cottage cheese
Juice of 1 small fresh lemon
1/2 small onion, chopped
1/4 cup fresh parsley, chopped
1/4 tsp. dry mustard powder
1/4 tsp. black pepper

Blend all of ingredients together in a blender. Let marinate in a covered container in refrigerator for at least 2 hours.

DIP 3:   **Spicy Tuna**

1 can (6 ounces) water-pack tuna, drained and rinsed
Juice of 1 small fresh lemon
1 tsp. minced garlic
1/2 medium onion, chopped
Few drops hot pepper sauce
1/2 - 1 tsp. curry powder
1/4 cup fresh parsley, chopped

Blend all ingredients together in blender, until almost smooth. Let marinate in refrigerator overnight.

DIP 4:   **Veggie Bean Dip**

 1 - 16 oz. can vegetarian baked beans
 1/2 medium onion, chopped
 Juice of 1 fresh lemon
 1 tsp. minced garlic
 1 tsp. dry mustard powder
 1/2 tsp. hot pepper sauce
 1/4 - 1/2 tsp. Worcestershire sauce
 1/4 tsp. black pepper
 1/2 tsp. Mrs. Dash

 Blend all of ingredients together in blender. Let marinate in refrigerator for at least 2 hours.

Note: 1.   To thicken any of above dips, use coffee grinder to grind raw oatmeal to a powder. Then add powder to mixture prior to marinating period.

            2.   All of the above dips make an excellent topping over baked potatoes, which have already been topped with steamed vegetables and Molly McButter.

            3.   **Bonus:** Adding ground oatmeal to a dip or spread increases the fiber content, as well.

Notes: _____

144

Seafood Dip / Seafood Spread

1/2 lb. imitation crabmeat, flaked
4 ounces lowfat cream cheese
1/2 cup plain, nonfat yogurt
1/2 medium onion, diced

1 - 2 tsp. Bragg's Liquid Aminos
1/8 - 1/4 tsp. hot pepper sauce
1 tbsp. prepared horseradish
Paprika

1. In a blender, blend the cream cheese and yogurt together.
2. In a bowl, thoroughly combine all of the ingredients, including the blended mixture.
3. Cover and refrigerate for at least 30 minutes. Sprinkle with paprika.

Note: Tuna, Salmon, Shrimp, or real Crabmeat can be substituted for the imitation crabmeat.

Nippy Dippy

1 can (16 ounces) black beans,
    drained and rinsed
2 medium cloves of garlic
1/2 medium onion, chopped

1/2 tsp. cumin
1/8 - 1/4 tsp. hot pepper sauce
Juice of 1 fresh lemon
Water, as needed

In a blender or Vita-Mix machine, blend all of the ingredients until smooth, about 1 minute. Only add water if necessary.

Hummus: Chickpea Dip / Chickpea Spread

1 can (16 ounces) chickpeas, drained
2 - 3 medium cloves garlic
2 tbsp. tahini
Juice of 1 fresh lemon

2 tbsp. tamari
3 tbsp. fresh parsley, chopped
1/4 tsp. cumin
1/8 - 1/4 tsp. hot pepper sauce

In a blender or Vita-Mix machine, blend all ingredients until smooth. Should be thick. Cover and refrigerate for at least 4 hours to meld the flavors.

Variation: For **Curried Chickpea Dip and Spread**, eliminate the tamari and cumin, and add 1 - 2 tsp. curry powder, 1 tsp. Spicy Mrs. Dash and 1 large tomato, diced. Blend all of the ingredients, except the tomatoes. Stir in tomatoes and chill as above.

Garlic Cheese Dip

1 cup nonfat cottage cheese
2 medium cloves of garlic
1 tbsp. all natural butter sprinkles

1 tsp. dried chives
1/8 - 1/4 tsp. fresh ground pepper

In a blender or Vita-Mix machine, blend all ingredients until smooth. Cover and refrigerate for at least 4 hours prior to serving.

Tangy Chili Dip

1 can (16 ounces) pinto beans
1 cup plain, nonfat yogurt
1/2 cup canned green chilis
1/2 medium onion, chopped

1/4 tsp. cumin
2 tbsp. Parmesan cheese
2 tsp. chili powder

In a blender or Vita-Mix machine, blend all ingredients until smooth. Cover and refrigerate for several hours prior to serving.

Notes:

Guacamole Dip

1 medium onion, chopped	1 tbsp. Bragg's Liquid Aminos
2 large cloves of garlic	1/8 - 1/4 tsp. hot pepper sauce
2 avocados	Juice of 1/2 fresh lemon
1/4 cup plain, nonfat yogurt	2 medium tomatoes. diced

In a blender or Vita-Mix machine, blend all ingredients, except the tomatoes, until smooth. In a bowl, mix the tomatoes into the blended mixture. Chill for at least 1 hour prior to serving. Garnish with chopped scallions and tomatoes.

Variation: For **Chickpea Guacamole Dip and Spread**, add 1 can (16 ounces) of chickpeas and an additional 1/2 cup of plain, nonfat yogurt to the mixture,   prior to blending all of the ingredients, except the tomatoes. For a chunkier consistency reduce the blending time. As above, *mix* the tomatoes in last.

Note: **Chickpeas** and **Garbanzo Beans** are the same thing!

Beans as Dips, Spreads or Dressings

1.   To make **Salad Dressings, Sauces or Sandwich Spreads,** simply adjust the amount of liquid in the recipe. Adding more liquid creates a thinner more dressing-like consistency. Eliminating some of the liquid creates a thicker consistency, which is more appropriate for a spread.

2.   For most dips, dressings and spreads which use beans as a base, experiment with flavors, substituting one type of bean for another in the recipe. For example, substitute black beans for chickpeas, or vice versa. Or substitute pinto beans or blackeyed peas for chickpeas or black beans. *The sky is the limit when you become adventurous with your taste sensations!*

Notes: _____

Cottage Cheese and Applesauce Spread

1/2 cup nonfat cottage cheese   1/2 tsp. cinnamon
1/2 cup applesauce, commercial   1/4 tsp. nutmeg
     or homemade*

1. Either mix all of the ingredients together for a more lumpy consistency, or blend together for a smoother consistency. (My preference is smooth, because it spreads more easily.)
2. After blending the mixture, let it sit for 30 - 60 minutes to blend the flavors.

Variation: Ricotta cheese can be substituted for the cottage cheese.

* See the recipe for homemade applesauce.

Makes 2 servings

Ricotta Cheese and Fruit Spread

1/2 cup ricotta cheese   1/2 medium banana
1 tbsp. unsulphured raisins or dates

In a blender or Vita-Mix machine, blend all ingredients together until smooth.

Variations:
1. Add 1 mango to the existing recipe.
2. Substitute 1 mango for the banana in the recipe.
3. Substitute with any fresh ripe fruit in season.
4. Substitute the dried fruit with 1/2 of a fresh, ripe avocado.
5. Substitute the ricotta cheese with nonfat cottage cheese.
6. Substitute the dried fruit in the recipe with dried apricots.
7. Eliminate the dried fruit in the recipe.

Makes 2 servings

Notes: _____

References and Resources

BOOKS: FOOD, NUTRITION AND FOOD SAFETY

■ Balch, J. & P. **Prescription for Nutritional Healing.** New York: Avery Publishing Group, 1990.

■ Barnard, N., M.D. **The Power of Your Plate.** Tennessee: Book Publishing Co., 1990.

■ Barnard, N., M.D. **Food for Life: How the New Four Food Groups Can Save Your Life.** New York: Crown Trade Paperbacks, 1994.

■ Brody, J. **Jane Brody's Nutrition Book.** New York: Bantam Books, Inc., 1987.

■ Brody, J. **Jane Brody's Good Food Book.** New York: Bantam Books, Inc., 1985.

■ Chopra, D., M.D. **Perfect Health.** New York: Harmony Books, 1990.

■ Connor, W., M.D. and S. **The New American Diet.** New York: Simon & Schuster, Inc., 1986.

■ Cousens, G., M.D. **Conscious Eating.** Vision Books International, 510 Fifth St., Santa Rosa, CA 95401, (707) 542-1440, 1992.

■ Frahm, A. & D. **Healthy Habits: 20 Simple Ways to Improve Your Health.** Pinon Press, P.O. box 35007, Colorado Springs, CO 80935, (719) 593-8694.

■ Goor, R. **Eater's Choice: A Food Lover's Guide to Lower Cholesterol.** Houghton Miflin, 1987.

■ Guste, R., Jr. **Louisiana Light.** W.W. Norton & Co., 1990.

■ Haas, E., M.D. **Staying Healthy with Nutrition.** Celestial Arts Publishing P.O. Box 7327, Berkeley, CA 94707, 1992.

■ Havala, S., R.D. **Simple, Lowfat & Vegetarian.** Maryland: The Vegetarian Resource Group, 1994.

■ Jacobson, M., Ph.D. **Safe Food: Eating Wisely in a Risky World.** Living Planet Press, 558 Rose Avenue, Venice, CA 90291, (213) 396-0188.

■ Jensen, B., M.D. **Foods That Heal.** New York: Avery Publishing Group, Inc., 1988.

- Jordan, P., R.N. **How the New Food Labels Can Save Your Life.** Michael Wiese Productions, 4354 Laurel Canyon Blvd., #234, Studio City, CA 91694, (818) 379-8799, 1994.

- Lappe, F. Moore. **Diet for a Small Planet.** New York; Ballantine Books, 10th Ed. 1982.

- Levenstein, M. **Everyday Cancer Risks and How to Avoid Them.** New York: Avery Publishing Group, 1992.

- McDougall, J. & M. **The McDougall Plan.** New Jersey: New Century Publishers, 1983.

- Nelson, D. **Food Combining Simplified.** D. Nelson, P.O. Box 2302, Santa Cruz, CA 95063. Also produces pocket cards and wall charts for easy reference.

- Null, G., Ph.D. **The 90's Healthy Body Book: How to Overcome the Effects of Pollution and Cleanse the Toxins from Your Body.** Florida: Health Communications, Inc., 1994.

- Ornish, D., M.D. **Eat More, Weigh Less.** New York: Harper Collins Publishers, Inc., 1993.

- Ornish, D., M.D. **Dr. Dean Ornish's Program for Reversing Heart Disease.** New York: Ballantine Books, 1990.

- Possick, K. **Consumer Alert Publications:** 1) **Antioxidants:** Halting the Disease Process in Your Family; 2) **Tired of Being Tried?** Tired of Being Sick? Just Fed Up?; and 3) **Why are You Poisoning Your Family?** Kare Possick, Box 86036, Madeira Beach, FL 33738, (813) 397-0202, 1994-95.

- Quillin, P., Ph.D. **Healing Nutrients.** New York: Random House, Inc., 1987.

- Quillin, P., Ph.D. **Beating Cancer with Nutrition.** The Nutrition Times Press, Inc., Box 700512, Tulsa, Ok 74170-0512, (918) 495-1137, 1994.

- Robbins, J. **Diet for a New World: May All Be Fed.** New York: Avon Books, 1992.

- Robbins, J. **Diet for a New America.** New Hampshire: Stillpoint Publishing, 1987.

- Robertson, L. **The New Laurel's Kitchen.** Ten Speed Press, 1987.

- Santillo, H. **Food Enzymes: The Missing Link to Radiant Health.** Hohm Press, 1987.

- Schechter, Steven, N.D. **Fighting Radiation and Chemical Pollutants with Foods, Herbs, & Vitamins.** Vitality, Ink, P.O. Box 294, Encinitas, CA 92024, (619) 943-8485, 1988.

■ Shelton, H. **Food Combining Made Easy.** San Antonio, TX: Willow Publishing, 1989.

■ Shuman, M.R. **Mediterranean Light.** New York: Bantam Books, Inc., 1989.

■ Simone, C. **Cancer and Nutrition.** New York: Avery Publishing Group, Inc., 1992.

■ Wasserman, D. **Simply Vegan.** The Vegetarian Resource Group, P.O. Box 1463, Baltimore, MD 21203, 1991.

■ Wigmore, A. **The Hippocrates Diet.** New Jersey: Avery Publishing Group, 1984.

PSYCHONEUROIMMUNOLOGY
STRESS MANAGEMENT, ATTITUDE, RELAXATION, IMAGERY

■ Achterberg, J. **Imagery in Healing.** Boston: Shambhala Publications, 1985.

■ Anderson, G. **The Cancer Conqueror.** Kansas City: Andrews & McMeel, 1988.

■ Anderson, G. **The Triumphant Patient.** Kansas City: Andrews & McMeel, 1992.

■ Benjamin, H., Ph.D. **From Victim to Victor.** New Your: Bantam Doubleday Dell Publishing Group, 1987.

■ Benson, H. **The Relaxation Response.** New York: William Morrow & Co., 1975.

■ Benson, H. **Your Maximum Mind: Changing Your Life by Changing the Way You Think.** New York: Random House, 1987.

■ Borysenko, J. Ph.D. **Guilt is the Teacher, Love is the Lesson.** New York: Warner Books, Inc., 1990.

■ Borysenko, J., Ph.D. **Minding the Body, Mending the Mind.** Massachusetts: Addison-Wesley Publishing Co., 1987.

■ Cousins, N. **Anatomy of an Illness as Perceived by a Patient: Reflections on Healing and Regeneration.** New York: W.W. Norton & Co., 1979.

■ Cousins, N. **Head First: The Biology of Hope.** New York: E.P. Dutton, 1989.

■ Dossey, L. **Recovering the Soul: A Scientific and Spiritual Search.** New York: Bantam Books, 1990.

■ Dossey, L. **Meaning of Medicine.** New York: Bantam Books, 1991.

■ Epstein, G. **Healing Visualizations: Creating Health Through Imagery.** New York: Bantam Books., 1989.

■ LeShan, L. **How to Meditate.** New York: Bantam Books, 1974.

■ LeShan, L. **Cancer as a Turning Point.** New York: E.P. Dutton, 1989.

■ Moyers, B. **Healing and The Mind.** New York: Bantam Doubleday Books, 1993.

■ Pelletier, K. **Mind as a Healer, Mind as a Slayer.** New York: Dell Publishing Co., 1977.

References and Resources (continued)

- Rosenberg, S.A. **The Transformed Cell: Unlocking the Mysteries on Cancer.** New York: Putnam Publishing Co., 1992.

- Seligman, M.E.P. **Learned Optimism: How to Change Your Mind and Your Life.** New York: Pocket Books, 1990.

- Selye, H. **The Stress of Life.** New York: McGraw-Hill, 1956.

- Siegel, B., M.D. **Love, Medicine and Miracles.** New York: Harper and Row, 1986.

- Siegel, B., M.D. **Peace, Love and Healing.** New York: Harper and Row, 1989.

- Simonton, O.C. & S. **Getting Well Again.** New York: Bantam Books, 1978.

- Simonton, O.C. & Henson, R. **The Healing Journey.** New York: Bantam Books, 1992.

- Storey, J. & M. **How-To Books for Country Living.** Do-It Yourself Bulletins, Books, Recipes, etc. Storey Communications, Inc., Dept. 72, P.O. Box 38, Pownal, Vermont 05261-9989; (800) 441-5700.

Notes: This is by no means an exhaustive book list. But it will assist you on the road to wellness. There is enough of a selection here that everyone should be able to find something from the list which is in line with his or her interest, or concern.

AUDIO AND VIDEO RENTALS

Apart from the books listed, many of the authors also offer taped versions of their books or programs, or of meditations for specific conditions. So if books are just not your thing, have no fear! Simply inquire about the availability of audio cassette programs, or video programs, by an author whose book title appeals to you.

Something that I have found to be of great value over the past two years, has been a membership with a company which sells and rents audio and video tapes by a mail order system. Instead of spending huge amounts of money buying every taped program that interests me, I simply rent it and *"try it before I buy it"*, at the rate of approximately one program per month. I get what I need from the program, playing it in the car, or at home when I'm relaxing, and then return it, and wait for the next program I have ordered to arrive. It has saved me tremendous amounts of money and has been a great way to avoid the clutter of a lot of programs taking up valuable shelf space. **After all, how many times have we bought an expensive cassette or video program, listened to it, or viewed it, only once, and then left it sitting on a shelf to collect dust until we gave it away or threw it away?**

The company I'm speaking of always has an up-to-date listing of programs available. And if you decide you want to buy a copy of a particular program you have listened to, members receive excellent discounts. For further information contact:

The Motivational Tape Company,
16760 Devonshire Street., #9
Granada Hills, California 91344
(818) 366-7500
Contact: Paul Arroyo

MAGAZINES, JOURNALS & NEWSLETTERS

American Fitness Magazine:
15250 Ventura Boulevard, Suite 310
Sherman Oaks, CA 91403
(800) 445-5950

Berkeley Wellness Letter:
P.O. Box 420148
Palm Coast, FL 32142
(904) 445-6414

Changes Magazine:
Changes
P.O. Box 609
Mount Morris, IL 61054-0609
(800) 998-0793

Consumer Reports on Health:
Consumers Union
Dept. GH, 101 Truman Ave.
Yonkers, N.Y. 10703-1057
(914) 378-2000

Coping Magazine:
2019 N. Carothers
Franklin, TN 37064

Eating Well Magazine:
P.O. Box 52919
Boulder, CO 80322-2919
(800) 678-0541

Health Magazine:
P.O. Box 56863
Boulder, CO 80322-6863
(800) 274-2522

HerbalGram:
American Botanical Council
P.O. Box 201660
Austin, TX 78720
(512) 331-8868

Natural Healing Newsletter:
FC&A Publishing
103 Clover Green
Peachtree City, GA 30269

Natural Health Magazine:
P.O. Box 57320
Boulder, CO 80322-7320

New Perspectives Magazine: P.O. Box 3208
Hemet, CA 92546
(909) 925-6117

Nutrition Action Health Letter: Center for Science in the Public Interest
1875 Connecticut Ave., N.W., Ste. 300
Washington, D.C. 20009-5728
(202) 332-9110

Obesity & Health Journal: Healthy Living Institute
402 South 14th St., Hettinger, ND 58639
(701) 567-2845

Tufts University Diet &
Nutrition Letter: P.O. Box 57857
Boulder, CO 80322-7857
(800) 274-7581

Vegetarian Journal: The Vegetarian Resource Group
P.O. Box 1463, Baltimore, MD 21203
(410) 366-8343

Vegetarian Gourmet: P.O. Box 10647,
Riverton, NJ 08076-0647

Vegetarian Times: P.O. Box 446
Mount Morris, IL 61054
(800) 435-9610

Veggie Life: P.O. Box 57159
Boulder, CO 80323

Yoga Journal: P.O. Box 469018
Escondido, CA 92046-9018
(800) 334-8152

Notes: Because a magazine or journal is listed here, does not mean that everything in the content of each will agree with the information contained within **"5 Minutes to Health"**. There is simply enough good information that warrants the magazine or journal being listed. It is up to you, as a discerning reader, to evaluate what is written and use only what will benefit your health to the maximum. For example, where recipes list ingredients, such as sweeteners and fats, not recommended, substitute with those included in your **"5 Minutes to Health"** shopping list.

ORGANIZATIONS & CENTERS FOR NUTRITION AND HEALTH

American Botanical Council:
P.O. Box 201660
Austin, TX 78720
(512) 331-8868

Ann Wigmore Foundation:
196 Commonwealth Ave.
Boston, MA 02116
(617) 267-9424

Center For Science in the
Public Interest:
1875 Connecticut Ave., N.W., Ste 300
Washington, D.C. 20009-5728
(202) 332-9110

Community Nutrition Institute:
2001 S. St., N.W., Ste 530
Washington, D.C. 20009
(202) 462-4700

Consumers Union:
101 Truman Avenue
Yonkers, New York 10703
(914) 378-2000

Creative Health Institute:
918 Union City Road
Union City, MI 49094
(517) 278-6260

Herb Research Foundation:
1007 Pearl St., Ste 200
Boulder, CO 80302
(303) 449-2265

Hippocrates Health Institute:
1443 Palmdale Court
West Palm Beach, FL 33411
(407) 471-8876

National Coalition to
Stop Food Irradiation:
P.O. Box 59-0488
San Francisco, CA 94159
(415) 566-2734

Optimum Health Institute
of San Diego:
6970 Central Avenue
Lemon Grove, CA 91945
(619) 464-3346

Physicians Committee for
Responsible Medicine:

P.O. Box 6322
Washington, D.C. 20015
(202) 686-2210

Public Voice for Food and
Health Policy:

1001 Connecticut Avenue, N.W., Ste 522
Washington, D.C. 20036
(202) 659-5930

Simonton Cancer Centers:

P.O. Box 623
Bridgeport, TX 76426
(800) 338-2360 or (817) 575-2420

and

15602 Sunset Blvd.
Pacific Palisades, CA 90272
(310) 459-4434

Vegetarian Nutrition Dietetic
Practice Group:

c/o The American Dietetic Association
216 West Jackson Blvd., Ste. 800
Chicago, IL 60606-6995

The Vegetarian Resource Group:

P.O. Box 1463, Baltimore, MD 21203
(410) 366-8343

INFORMATION, REFERRALS, DIRECTORIES

The American Association of Naturopathic Physicians:
P.O. Box 20386
Seattle, WA 98102
(206) 323-7610

American Cancer Society:
1599 Clifton Road, N.E.
Atlanta, GA 30329
(800) 227-2345

American College of Advances in Medicine:
231 Verdugo Dr., Ste. 204
Laguna Hills, CA 92653
(714) 583-7666

American Holistic Medical Association:
4101 Lake Boone Trail, Ste. 201
Raleigh, NC 27607
(919) 787-5146

The American Institute for Cancer Research:
1759 R St., N.W.
Washington, D.C. 20069
(800) 843-8114 or (202) 328-7744

The American Massage Therapy Association:
820 Davis St., Ste 100
Evanston, IL 60201
(708) 864-0123

Association for Research of Childhood Cancer:
P.O. Box 251
Buffalo, NY 14225
(716) 681-4433

Cancer Control Society:
2043 North Berendo St.
Los Angeles, CA 90027
(213) 663-7801

Cancer Information Service National Cancer Institute:
Boy Scout Bldg., R.340
Bethesda, MD 20892
(800) 4-CANCER or (301) 496-8664

Commission for Freedom of Choice in Medicine:
1180 Walnut Avenue
Chula Vista, CA 92011
(800) 227-4473

Intl. Academy of Nutrition &
Preventative Medicine:

P.O. Box 18433
Asheville, NC 28814
(704) 258-3243

The International Foundation
for Homeopathy:

2366 Eastlake Ave. E., Ste. 329
Seattle, WA 98102
(206) 324-8230

International Holistic Center, Inc.:

1042 Willow Creek Road, A111-151
Prescott, AZ 86301
(520) 771-1742

International Health Information
Institute:

14417 Chase St., Ste. 432
Panorama City, CA 91402

National Center for Environmental
Health Strategies:

1100 Rural Ave.
Voorhees, NJ 08043
(609) 429-5358

National Self-Help Clearinghouse:

25 West 43rd St., Room 620
New York, New York 10036

National Women's Health Network:

1325 G St., N.W.
Washington, D.C. 20005
(202) 347-1140

Nutrition Education Association, Inc.:

3647 Glen Haven
Houston, TX 77025
(713) 665-2946

The Health Resource:

209 Katherine Drive
Conway, AR 72032
(501) 329-5272

Wellness Community National
Headquarters:

1235 5th St., Santa Monica, CA 90401
(800) PRO-HOPE or (310) 393-1425

World Research Foundation:

15300 Ventura Blvd., Ste. 405
Sherman Oaks, CA 91403
(818) 907-5483

Notes: Some of the above organizations, institutes, centers, and services charge a nominal fee for their services and information. It is wise to inquire as to the cost, if any, prior to receiving what they have to offer. This saves confusion and prevents embarrassment later.

GOVERNMENT CONTACTS

Community Nutrition Institute:	1146 19th St., N.W. Washington, D.C. 20036
Consumer Information Center:	Department 609K Pueblo, CO 81009
Department of Agriculture Human Nutrition Info Service:	6505 Belcrest Rd. Hyattsville, MD 20782 (301) 436-8617
Department of Agriculture Food and Nutrition Service:	3101 Park Center Drive Alexandria, VA 22302 (703) 756-3276
Environmental Protection Agency (EPA):	401 M St., S.W. Washington, D.C. 20460 (202) 382-2090 EPA Safe Drinking Water Hotline: (800) 426-4791 or (202) 382-5533
Food and Drug Administration (FDA):	Dept. of Health and Human Services 5600 Fishers Lane Rockville, MD 20857 (301) 443-3170
National Marine Fisheries Service:	Dept. of Commerce 1335 East-West Highway Silver Spring, MD 20910 (301) 427-2358
United States Department of Agriculture (USDA):	14th St. and Independence Ave., S.W. Washington, D.C. 20250 (202) 447-2791
USDA Food Safety and Inspection Service (FSIS):	FSIS Consumer Inquiries / USDA Washington, D.C. 20250 (202) 472-4485 Meat and Poultry Hotline: (800) 535-4555

Organic Farmers: Mail Order Service

Though many stores in large cities carry certified organic produce and grains, these products may be very difficult to find in smaller centers and remote areas. As there are several sources for listings of organic farmers who mail order to the general public, I am not including a long list here. However, to assist you in this search I will include some sources of such listings.

Safe Food: Eating Wisely in a Risky World:

A book written by Jacobson, M.F., Lefferts, L.Y., and Garland, A.W. For this book and a list of other valuable resources, contact the **Center for Science in the Public Interest,** 1875 Connecticut Ave., N.W., Suite 300, Washington, D.C. 20009-5728, or call (202) 332-9110.

1995 National Organic Directory:

Though not specifically targeted to the general public, it is an excellent and comprehensive resource, listing farmers and wholesalers who actually do mail order to such an audience. For information on how to order this directory, contact the **Community Alliance with Family Farmers,** P.O. Box 464, Davis, CA 95617, or call (800) 852-3832.

Charan Springs Farm:

Owned by Michael Limacher. For some of the most flavorful organic produce available overnight by mail order, at very reasonable prices, write to **Charan Springs Farm,** Route #1, Box 521, Cambria, CA 93428, or call (805) 927-8289. And for anyone who wants a magical break from their daily routine, stay at one of the farm's secluded, well-equipped cabins. The combination of the all-natural food and the peaceful, unspoiled environment promotes the total rejuvenation of both body and mind!

Products and Equipment

The following is by no means an exhaustive list of healthy products and equipment. It is simply a summation of some of the items which have been mentioned throughout this book, but which may be, at this time, unavailable or difficult to find, in the regular marketplace. The sources accompanying each of the items listed, will provide you with information on how to order their products, or an outline of the retail locations nearest you which carry their products.

Note: Because a company's products are mentioned here, does not indicate that **5 Minutes to Health** *exclusively endorses that specific brand of that particular product. It is simply a base from which to begin your own research.*

REMEMBER! Be adventurous! Try new foods, seasonings and condiments!

Seasoning

All-Natural Flavor Sprays

Tryson House
A Div. of Par-Way/Tryson Companies
107 Bolte Lane
St. Clair, MO 63077
(800) 222-6820

Bragg's Liquid Aminos

For information and recipes:
Live Food Products, Inc.
Box 7, Santa Barbara, CA 93102

Dr. Bronner's Mineral Bouillon

For information and recipes:
All-One-God-Faith, Inc.
Box 28, Escondido, CA 92033

Gayelord Hauser's All Natural Vegetable Broth Powder

For information and recipes:
Gayelord Hauser Products
P.O. Box 09398
Milwaukee, WI 53209

Molly McButter

For nutrition information and recipes:
(800) 622-3274

Mrs. Dash, Spicy Mrs. Dash,
Herbs, Spices, Sauces

For information on low-sodium diets, recipes,
diet tips:
Alberto Culver Co.
(800) 622-DASH (622-3274)

NOH of Hawaii Seasoning Mixes

NOH Foods of Hawaii
P.O. Box 7513
Torrance, CA 90504

Real Salt (Natural Mineral Salt)

For information:
American Orsa Inc.
P.O. Box 189
Redmont, UT 84652
(801) 529-7487 or (800) 367-7258

Take-5 Vegetable Refresher
Powder: a juice or a seasoning

For information and uses:
Custom Foods Inc.
Vernon, CA 90058
(619) 544-6442

.Yamaka All Purpose Sauce

For information and recipes:
Real Fresh Cookin'
P.O. Box 90728
Honolulu, HI 96835

Protein Powder and Spirulina

Spirulina Powder

For nutritional information and ideas for use:
Nutrex Hawaiian Spirulina Pacifica
NHI Nutrex, Inc.
Kailua-Kona, HI 96745
(215) 584-1252

Super-Green Pro-96 Protein Powder

Nature's Life
Cypress, CA 90630

Wholegrain Products

All Natural Baked Granola

For information:
Bowl 'A Granola; Rochelle Collins
P.O. Box 571
San Anselmo, CA 94979
(415) 459-2543

Barbara's Nature's Choice Organic Whole Grain Products and Snacks

For nutrition and product information:
Barbara's Bakery, Inc.
3900 Cypress Drive
Petaluma, CA 94954

Health Valley Cereals, Cookies, Crackers, Snacks, Soups, Meals

For nutrition information, diet tips and charts:
Health Valley Products
16100 Foothill Blvd.
Irwindale, CA 91706-7811
(818) 334-3241

Jammers Cookies, 7-Grainers Crackers, Fat Free and Whole Grain

For nutrition and product information:
Auburn Farms, Inc.
P.O. Box 348180
Sacramento, CA 95834

Natural Stone Ground Wholegrains, Bulk Grains, Cereals, Meals, Seeds, Seasoning Mixes and Beans

For information on mail order purchases and retailers:
Bob's Red Mill Natural Foods, Inc.
5209 S.E. International Way
Milwaukee, OR 97222
(503) 654-3215

Nine Grain Wholewheat Bread

For information:
Great Harvest Bread Co.
1808 Garnet Avenue, Pacific Plaza II
Pacific Beach
San Diego, CA 92109-3352
(619) 272-3521

Products and Equipment (continued)

Cheese and Meat

Healthy Choice Cheeses, Meats, Canned Products, etc.

For nutrition information and recipes:
Con Agra Consumer Affairs
Dept. BC, P.O. Box 3768
Omaha, NE 68103-0768
(800) 323-9980

Tofu

Cheese Substitute: Vegan Rella, Tofu Rella, Almond Rella and Zero-Fat Rella

For nutrition information, recipes and retailers:
Sharon's Finest Healthy Alternatives
P.O. Box 5020
Santa Rosa, CA 95402-5020
(707) 576-7050

Silken Tofu, Mori-Nu Brand

For information, recipes, cookbooks, videos:
Morinaga Nutritional Foods, Inc.
2050 W. 190th Street, Suite 110
Torrance, CA 90504
(800) NOW-TOFU (669-8638)

Tofu, Reduced Fat

For questions and information on selection:
Mycal Group Soy Production Division
(310) 791-0010

Soymilk

Soymilk, Endensoy

For nutrition information and recipes:
Eden Foods, 701 Tecumseh Road
Clinton, MI 49236
(800) 248-0320

Soymilk, Vitasoy

For nutrition information and recipes:
Vitasoy, Inc., 99 Park Lane
Brisbane, CA 94005
(415) 467-8888

Products and Equipment (continued)

Fat Replacements

Dried Plums in Baking
(Dried Plum Puree)

For fat replacement information and recipes:
California Prune Board
P.O. Box 10157
Pleasanton, CA 94588-0157
(800) 729-5992

Just Like Shortenin'
(a nonfat shortening substitute)

For information and recipes:
The PlumLife Company
15 Orchard Park, Suite 15
Madison, CT 06440
(203) 245-5993

Teas

Celestial Seasonings Herb Teas

For information on ordering and local retailers:
1780 55th Street
Boulder, CO 80301-2799

Good Earth Natural Herb Teas

For information on ordering and local retailers:
Wildcraft Herbs
831 Almar Avenue
Santa Cruz, CA 95060

Coffee Substitute

Coffee Substitute, Antioxidant
(Raja's Cub)

For information and catalog of herbal products:
MAPI
P.O. Box 49667
Colorado Springs, CO 80949-9667
(800) 255-8332, ext. 170

Meal-in-a-Cup

Soups and Meals, in a Cup
Dehydrated, Natural

For information on nutrition and retailers:
    Pacific Foods of Oregon, Inc.
    Tualatin, OR 97062

Soups and Meals, in a Cup
Dehydrated, Natural

For information on nutrition and retailers:
    Fantastic Foods, Inc.
    Petaluma, CA 94954

Other

Pomi Chopped Tomatoes

Only ingredient: **Tomatoes**
Parmalat U.S.A. Corp.
Hasbrouck Hts., NJ 07604

Equipment

Vita-Mixer and Total
Nutrition Center

For information, recipe books and videos, etc.:
Vita Mix Corporation
8615 Usher Road
Cleveland, OH 44138-2199
(800) VITAMIX (848-2649)

Index

S

T

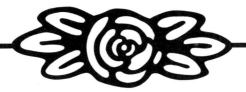

The Dilemma

To laugh is to risk appearing a fool.
To weep is to risk appearing sentimental.
To reach out for another is to risk involvement.
To expose feelings is to risk rejection.
To place your dreams before the crowd is to risk ridicule.
To love is to risk not being loved in return.
To go forward in the face of overwhelming odds is to risk failure.
But risks must be taken because the greatest hazard in life is to risk nothing.
The person who risks nothing does nothing, has nothing, is nothing.
He may avoid suffering and sorrow,
but he cannot learn, feel, change, grow or have.
Chained by his certitudes, he is a slave.
He has forfeited his freedom.
Only a person who takes risks is free.

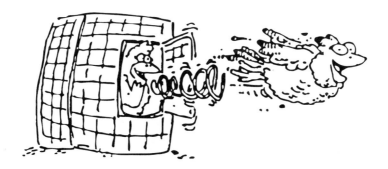

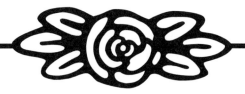

"Hugging"

No movable parts
No batteries to wear out
No monthly payments
No insurance requirements
Non-taxable
Non-polluting
Low energy consumption
High energy yield
Inflation proof
Hugging is healthy
It relieves tension
It combats depression
It reduces stress
It improves blood circulation
It is invigorating
It is rejuvenating
It elevates self-esteem
It generates good will
It has no unpleasant side effects
It is nothing less than a miracle drug
It will cure whatever ails you
and, of course, Fully Returnable

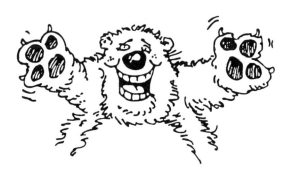